COLOUR GUIDE

Sexually Transmitted Infections

A. McMillan MD FRCP
Royal Infirmary of Edinburgh
The Lothian University Hospitals NHS Trust, UK

G. R. Scott MB ChB FRCP (Edin)
Royal Infirmary of Edinburgh
The Lothian University Hospitals NHS Trust, UK

SECOND EDITION

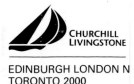

CHURCHILL
LIVINGSTONE

EDINBURGH LONDON N
TORONTO 2000
SYDNEY

D0242476

CHURCHILL LIVINGSTONE
An imprint of Harcourt Publishers Limited

© Harcourt Publishers Limited 2000

◢◢ is a registered trademark of Harcourt
Publishers Limited.
The right of A. McMillan and G. R. Scott to be
identified as authors of this work has been
asserted by them in accordance with the
Copyright, Designs and Patents Act 1988

First published as Colour Aids to Sexually
Transmitted Diseases 1991
First Colour Guide edition 2000

ISBN 0443 06229 3

British Library Cataloguing in Publication Data
A catalogue record for this book is available from
the British Library

**Library of Congress Cataloging in Publication
Data**
A catalog record for this book is available from
the Library of Congress

Note
Medical knowledge is constantly
changing. As new information
becomes available, changes in
treatment, procedures, equipment
and the use of drugs become
necessary. The authors and the
publishers have, as far as it is
possible, taken care to ensure
that the information given in this
text is accurate and up-to-date.
However, readers are strongly
advised to confirm that the
information, especially with
regard to drug usage, complies
with the latest legislation and
standards of practice.

The
publisher's
policy is to use
**paper manufactured
from sustainable forests**

Printed in China
SWTC/01

Commissioning Editor:
Michael Parkinson
Project Development Manager:
Siân Jarman
Project Manager: Frances Affleck
Design Direction: Erik Bigland

Acknowledgements

We gratefully acknowledge the generosity of the following individuals in providing slides from their own collections: Professor J. A. A. Hunter and colleagues, Department of Dermatology, University of Edinburgh; Professor C. I. Phillips, formerly Department of Ophthalmology, University of Edinburgh; Professor V. N. Sehgal, Delhi; Drs H. Young, J. F. Peutherer, I. W. Smith, Department of Clinical Microbiology, University of Edinburgh; Dr J. D. Oriel, Consultant Physician, formerly University College Hospital, London; Dr E. M. C. Dunlop, formerly Consultant Physician, Whitechapel Clinic, London; Dr J. P. Ackers, Department of Medical Protozoology, London School of Hygiene and Tropical Medicine; Dr D. Wray, Department of Oral Medicine, Glasgow University; Dr D. H. H. Robertson, formerly Consultant Physician, Department of Genito-Urinary Medicine, Royal Infirmary of Edinburgh; Dr J. G. McKenna, Consultant Physician, Sexual Health Services, Raigmore Hospital, Inverness; Dr G. Morrison, Consultant Physician, Department of Genitourinary Medicine, Plymouth; Dr R. Brettle, Regional Infectious Diseases Unit, Edinburgh.

  We gratefully acknowledge the help of the Department of Medical Photography, Royal Infirmary of Edinburgh and our secretary Mrs E. J. Whittaker.

Contents

The management of sexually transmitted infections (STIs) is generally undertaken within sexual health clinics or departments of genitourinary medicine. Attendance is voluntary, confidentiality is assured and treatment is free.

In addition to the management of STIs, many clinics offer a range of sexual health services, including contraception and psycho-sexual counselling.

Reasons for attendance at a clinic (Fig. 1)

Self-referral: for example, the patient noticed anogenital symptoms or is symptomless but perceives that he or she has been at risk of infection.

Result of partner notification: when an individual is identified as having an STI, the person who is the likely source of infection and any subsequent sexual partners should be invited to attend for investigation and, if necessary, treatment.

Confidentiality is of paramount importance and as thus, clinic records are stored within the clinic and are available only to the staff of that clinic. At reception, each new patient is given a unique number that is used instead of a name on the forms that accompany specimens sent to different laboratories, thereby safeguarding anonymity. If the person has attended as a contact of a patient with an STI, no information is given about the partner by the clinic staff.

Role of the health adviser

Partner notification is an integral part of the control of STIs. This is usually undertaken by a health adviser within the sexual health clinic. In addition, the health adviser (Fig. 2) has a major role in educating the public about risk reduction for all STIs, and this is undertaken both within the clinics and in the community, for example in schools.

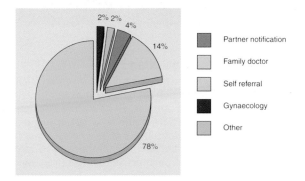

Fig. 1 Means of referral to a GUM clinic.

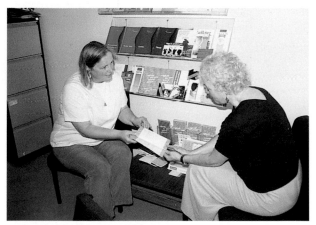

Fig. 2 Health adviser and patient.

Heterosexual man

A specific history should be taken to elicit any symptoms such as dysuria that the individual may not have recognised as being those of an STI. Notes should be made of whether or not he has a regular sexual partner and when he last had sex with her. In addition it is important to ask about other sexual partners within the preceding 6 months, and, if relevant, when sex with these partners occurred. He should be asked specifically if he has been told by a sexual partner that she has an infection. The use of barrier methods of contraception with any partner should be asked about. The use of any antimicrobial therapy within the preceding month should be noted. A past history of an STI should be recorded, and, if he has travelled outwith the UK within the preceding 6 months (Fig. 3), notes should be made of any sexual contact with local inhabitants, and if so, if condoms were used.

Homosexual man

The history taking is as above, but he should be asked about his sexual practices so that the appropriate investigations can be performed. He should be asked if he has insertive or receptive oral-genital sex, oral-anal sex, or anal intercourse. He should be asked specifically about anorectal symptoms such as persistent diarrhoea, anal discharge, anal bleeding and painful defaecation. It is important to note whether he has been vaccinated against hepatitis A and B.

Heterosexual woman

The details in the sexual history do not differ significantly from those described above for the heterosexual man. Notes should be made, however, of the date of her last menstrual period and the length of the cycle. The method of contraception used, if any, and an obstetric history should be recorded.

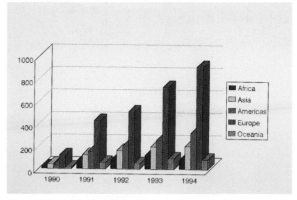

Fig. 3 An increasing number of men who attended sexual health clinics between 1990 and 1994 gave a history of sexual contact abroad with local people. (Data for men in Scotland 1990–1994.)

Heterosexual man

The extent of the physical examination will be determined by the history of the individual. For example, if the man has had a skin rash, as may occur in syphilis and HIV infection, it is important to undertake a general examination in addition to that of the anogenital area.

- Take material for culture for *Neisseria gonorrhoeae* from the tonsils or tonsillar fossae if there is a history of risk through oral-genital sex.
- Inspect the pubic area for *Pthirus pubis*.
- Examine the genito-crural folds.
- Palpate the inguinal lymph nodes and note enlargement with or without tenderness.
- Palpate the testes and epididymis.
- Examine the shaft of the penis for lesions such as herpes (Fig. 4) and scabetic papules (Fig. 5).
- Retract prepuce, if present, and look for lesions such as warts.
- Examine urethral meatus for urethral discharge; always evert the lips of the meatus to identify warts.
- Obtain material from the distal 5 cm of the urethra for Gram-stained smear microscopy using an inoculating loop and culture for *N. gonorrhoeae*.
- Examine perineum, perianal region and anus for example for warts.
- Examine urine for 'threads' (casts of the paraurethral glands) whose presence may indicate subacute urethritis.
- Send a 20 ml sample of urine to the microbiology laboratory for the detection of chlamydial DNA, or, using a cotton wool-tipped ENT swab, collect urethral material for detection of chlamydial DNA or antigen or for culture.
- Take blood for serological tests for syphilis, and, if indicated (p. 51), for hepatitis B surface antigen.
- Carry out HIV antibody test, if requested, and *only after appropriate counselling*.

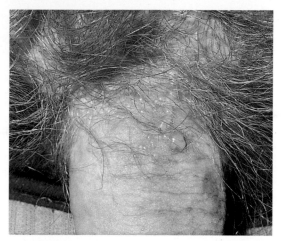

Fig. 4 Herpetic vesicles on shaft of penis.

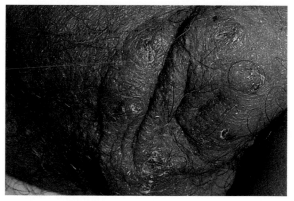

Fig. 5 Scabetic papules on scrotum.

Homosexual man

The physical examination is as that for the heterosexual man, but if there is a history of receptive anal intercourse, a proctoscope, lightly lubricated with KY jelly, should be passed and the distal rectum and anal canal inspected (Fig. 6).

The additional microbiological tests that should be undertaken are as follows:

- Pharyngeal culture for *N. gonorrhoeae* in every case.
- Using a cotton wool-tipped applicator stick that is inserted about 3 cm into the anal canal, obtain material for culture for *N. gonorrhoeae*.
- In addition, if there are symptoms or signs of proctitis (Fig. 7), take rectal specimens with a cotton wool-tipped applicator stick for culture for herpes simplex virus and *Chlamydia trachomatis*.
- If there is a history of diarrhoea, obtain a stool sample for culture for bacterial pathogens such as *Campylobacter* spp. and microscopy for trophozoites and/or cysts of the pathogenic protozoa *Giardia intestinalis*, *Cryptosporidium* spp. and, if there is a history of travel to tropical countries or sexual contact with an individual who has recently visited such areas, *Entamoeba histolytica*.
- If there is pruritus ani, make a sticky tape strip preparation and examine microscopically for eggs of *Enterobius vermicularis* (threadworm).
- Serological tests for hepatitis B, including test for surface and core antibodies against that virus (if there is no immunity, offer vaccination).
- Serological tests for specific IgG against hepatitis A virus (if there is no immunity, offer vaccination).
- Discuss HIV infection and, after counselling, offer HIV antibody test.

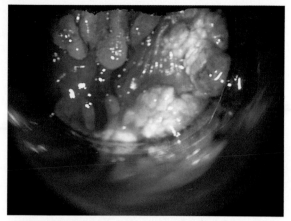

Fig. 6 Warts within anal canal of a homosexual man.

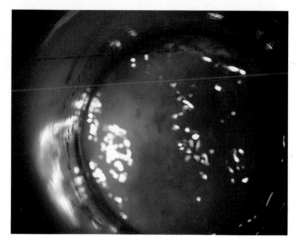

Fig. 7 Gonococcal proctitis.

Heterosexual woman

This physical examination should be performed with the woman in the semi-lithotomy position on a couch in a warm and well-lit room. Male doctors must have a chaperone.

- If the woman has been at risk of pharyngeal gonorrhoea, take material from the tonsils or tonsillar fossae for culture for the gonococcus.
- Inspect and palpate the abdomen for tenderness, guarding and masses.
- Inspect the pubic area for *P. pubis*, warts and molluscum contagiosum (Fig. 8).
- Palpate the inguinal lymph nodes, and note enlargement and tenderness.
- Inspect the labia majora, e.g. for warts or candidiasis (Fig. 9).
- Examine the labia minora and, after gently wiping with a cotton wool ball, the introitus. Look particularly for warts and the lesions of genital herpes (Fig. 10).
- Using a cotton wool-tipped applicator stick, take material from the urethra for Gram-smear microscopy and culture for *N. gonorrhoeae*.
- Palpate the greater vestibular glands, and note the character of the expressed secretions. In bartholinitis mucopus exudes from the orifices of the gland ducts.
- Prepare and examine microscopically a Gram-stained smear of any exudate from the ducts and culture for *N. gonorrhoeae*.
- Pass a speculum and examine the walls of the vagina. Note the character of any vaginal discharge, e.g. that associated with candidiasis is curdy and adheres to the vaginal walls.
- Using narrow-range pH paper held in a pair of forceps, measure the pH of the secretions in the posterior vaginal fornix (avoid the alkaline cervical secretions); in bacterial vaginosis pH ≥ 5.0.
- Examine microscopically a saline-mount preparation of material obtained from the posterior vaginal fornix with a cotton wool-tipped applicator stick for *Trichomonas vaginalis*, fungal hyphae and 'clue cells' of bacterial vaginosis.
- Examine microscopically a Gram-stained smear of material similarly obtained from the posterior fornix for 'clue cells' and hyphae of *Candida* spp.

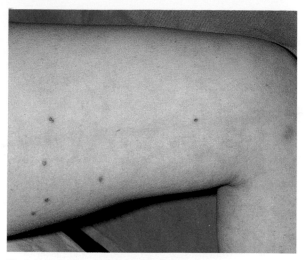

Fig. 8 Molluscum contagiosum on a woman's thigh.

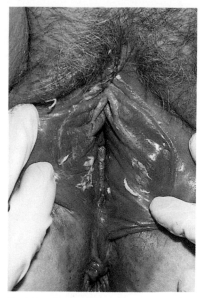

Fig. 9 Candidal vulvitis.

Heterosexual woman (contd)

- Note the appearance of the ectocervix and the character of any discharge from the endocervical canal; ulceration caused by herpes simplex virus may be seen (Fig. 11), and, in chlamydial infection, there may be a mucopurulent discharge.
- If the woman, aged 21 years or over, has not had a cervical smear taken within the preceding 3 years, undertake this, using an Ayre's or similar spatula *before* taking the endocervical specimens detailed below.
- Using a cotton wool-tipped applicator stick, take material from the endocervical canal for Gram-smear microscopy and culture for *N. gonorrhoeae*.
- Using a cotton wool-tipped applicator stick, take material from the endocervical canal for either (a) the detection of chlamydial DNA by PCR or LCR, or (b) culture for *C. trachomatis* (in 2SP transport medium), or (c) the detection of chlamydial antigens by EIA. The examination of urine by PCR or LCR for chlamydial DNA may conveniently replace the taking of genital material for microbiological examination.
- Inspect the perineum, perianal region and anus for lesions such as warts.
- Pass a cotton wool-tipped applicator stick about 3 cm into the anal canal, withdraw and plate out on MNYC medium for culture for *N. gonorrhoeae*.
- If there are anorectal symptoms, pass a proctoscope and examine the anal canal and distal rectum.
- Perform a bimanual vaginal examination looking for adnexal tenderness or swellings.
- If there is a risk of pregnancy, perform a test on urine.
- Take a blood sample for serological tests for syphilis (see above).
- If the woman is at risk of hepatitis B virus infection, undertake serological screening as above. If there is a risk of continuing exposure to that virus (p. 51) offer vaccination if she lacks immunity.
- Discuss HIV, and if requested after counselling, obtain blood for HIV antibody testing.

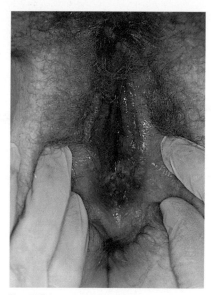

Fig. 10 Primary genital herpes.

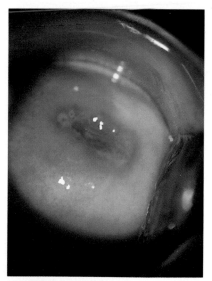

Fig. 11 Herpetic cervicitis.

4 / Urethritis in men

Presenting complaint

Urethral discharge (Fig. 12) and/or dysuria.
Additional features such as nocturia, urgency and fever should suggest the possibility of cystitis or prostatitis. A careful sexual history should be obtained.

Examination

Check for signs of other STIs. Examine the scrotal contents for signs of epididymo-orchitis. Examine the penis for warts or ulceration.

Collection of specimens

A plastic loop is used. Material for culture is plated directly onto a selective medium, e.g. MNYC. When direct plating is impracticable, specimens should be placed in a suitable transport medium, such as Amies. A first-voided urine specimen should be examined for chlamydial nucleic acids by PCR or LCR or urethral material for culture (sent in 2SP transport medium), DNA detection or for enzyme immunoassay should be obtained by passing a cotton wool-tipped ENT swab 2–4 cm into the urethra, rotating, and then withdrawing.

Diagnosis

A heat-fixed smear of exudate should be Gram-stained and examined by light microscopy. If Gram-negative diplococci (GNDC) are seen, a presumptive diagnosis of gonococcal urethritis (GU) is made, although this should always be confirmed by culture.
As microscopy will be negative in 10% of cases of GU, material for culture should be sent in every case. Non-gonococcal urethritis (NGU) is diagnosed if there are no GNDC, but >5–10 pus cells per high power field (×1000). If fewer pus cells are seen, or if 'threads' are seen in the urine (p. 5), the patient should be asked to return for an early morning smear, having held his urine overnight. Routine testing for chlamydiae is to be encouraged as this will occasionally yield positive results in the absence of significant numbers of pus cells. A two-glass urine test is routinely performed to differentiate anterior urethritis (Fig. 13) from posterior urethral inflammation.

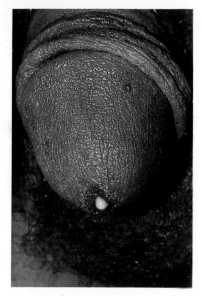

Fig. 12 Urethral discharge.

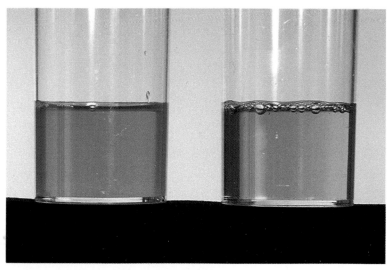

Fig. 13 Two-glass urine test to detect acute anterior urethritis.

The normal vaginal discharge is composed of secretions from the upper genital tract, cervical glands, the vagina (Figs 14 & 15), Bartholin's glands, and the periurethral, sebaceous and apocrine glands of the vulva.

Causes

Physiological causes
Secretions increase during ovulation, immediately before menstruation, during sexual arousal and during pregnancy. A white vaginal discharge may be noted during the first 10 d of life and for about a year before the onset of the menarche. In adult women anxiety, frequent erotic stimulation, the use of the oral contraceptive and cervical ectropion may be causes.

Infections
These include:
1. *Neisseria gonorrhoeae*.
2. *Chlamydia trachomatis*.
3. *Trichomonas vaginalis*.
4. *Candida* spp.
5. Bacterial vaginosis.
6. Warts caused by human papilloma virus.
7. Herpes simplex virus (HSV).

Other causes
1. Retained foreign bodies such as tampons.
2. Chemical vaginitis (Figs 16 & 17) such as from antiseptic use.
3. Secondary infection of vaginal and cervical tears.
4. Neoplasm that may be benign (cervical polyps) or malignant.

Diagnosis

A correct diagnosis depends on the taking of a careful history, a proper examination of the lower genital tract, and the appropriate microbiological investigations. In all cases the urine should be tested for glycosuria.

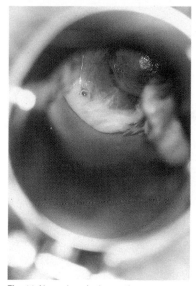

Fig. 14 Normal vaginal secretion.

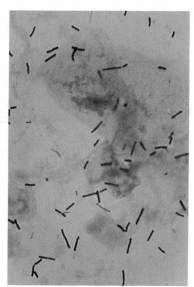

Fig. 15 Gram-stained smear of normal vaginal flora.

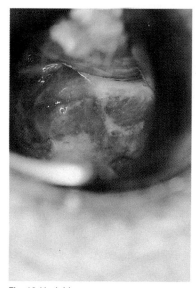

Fig. 16 Vaginitis.

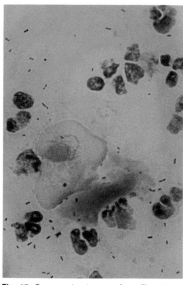

Fig. 17 Gram-stained smear from Fig. 16.

Causes and diagnosis

Bacterial infections
1. Syphilis diagnosed by dark-field microscopy or direct immunofluorescence and serology.
2. Chancroid diagnosed by Gram-smear microscopy and by culture of *Haemophilus ducreyi*.
3. Lymphogranuloma venereum diagnosed by culture of *C. trachomatis* or serology.
4. Granuloma inguinale diagnosed by Giemsa-stained smear microscopy or biopsy.
5. Pyogenic infection (Fig. 18) diagnosed by bacterial culture.
6. Tuberculosis (rare) diagnosed by biopsy or culture.

Viral infections
1. HSV diagnosed by culture (send specimen in Hank's viral transport medium – Fig. 19) or serology (primary infection only).
2. Herpes zoster: dermatomal distribution; diagnosis by culture.

Protozoal infestation
E. histolytica (rare): histological diagnosis.

Multisystem conditions
1. Erythema multiforme.
2. Behçets' syndrome.
3. Fixed drug eruptions.

Other causes
1. Chemical irritation with a history of contact.
2. Trauma: diagnosis made on history.
3. Malignancy: histological diagnosis.

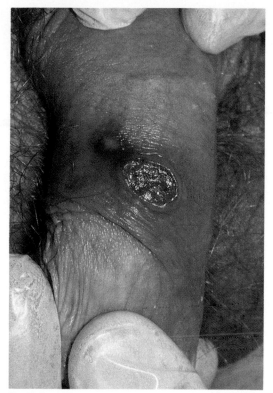

Fig. 18 Pyogenic genital ulcer.

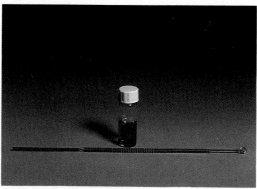

Fig. 19 Hank's viral transport medium.

7 / Non-specific genital infection

Aetiology

C. trachomatis causes 50–70% of cases of non-specific genital infection (NSGI) which in males is referred to as NGU (Fig. 20). *C. trachomatis* may be divided immunologically into a number of serotypes (serovars). Types A, B and C are associated with the ocular infection trachoma, types L 1–3 are associated with lymphogranuloma venereum, whereas the oculogenital serovars D–K are associated with NGU. The role of other organisms is less certain, but *Ureaplasma urealyticum*, *Mycoplasma genitalium*, and *Bacteroides* spp. may account for 10–20%. Occasional cases are due to infection with HSV, *T. vaginalis* and coliforms. In a significant proportion no organism is identified.

Epidemiology

NSGI is three times as common as gonococcal infection in the UK, with similar prevalence rates worldwide. Precise epidemiological observation has been hampered by difficulties in diagnosing chlamydial infection. The use of PCR or LCR for the detection of chlamydial nucleic acids in urine samples, however, permits wider screening for infection than has hitherto been possible.

Clinical features

In males
Chlamydial infection is symptomless in at least 25% of cases. In the remainder, and in cases of non-chlamydial NGU, the prepatent period is 1–4 weeks, following which a mucoid or mucopurulent discharge and/or dysuria develops. Symptoms are usually less marked than with gonococcal urethritis, but there is considerable overlap and differentiation on clinical grounds alone is not advised. Chlamydial infection of the rectum is usually symptomless.

Complications: the most important is epididymo-orchitis, of which chlamydiae are the commonest cause in young sexually active men. Auto-inoculation may result in conjunctivitis (Fig. 21). Reiter's syndrome is discussed on pp. 25–29. ➡

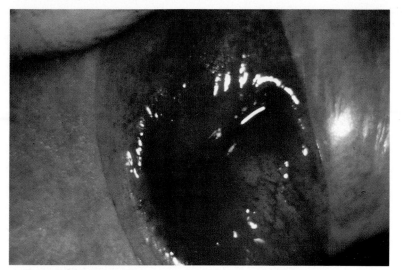

Fig. 20 Non-gonococcal urethritis.

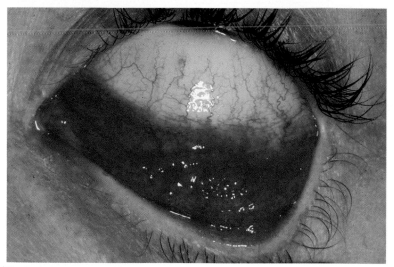

Fig. 21 Chlamydial conjunctivitis.

In females
Chlamydial infection of the cervix (Fig. 22) is usually symptomless, although examination may reveal a follicular or 'cobblestone' appearance. About one-third of patients complain of increased vaginal discharge. Urethral infection, present in more than 20% of cases, may result in dysuria and/or urinary frequency. Ascending infection may result in salpingitis for which chlamydiae are the single most common cause, accounting for approximately 30% of cases admitted to gynaecology units. The abdominal pain and degree of systemic upset are usually less marked than with gonococcal salpingitis. Spillage of infected material from the salpinges with transcoelomic spread to the liver capsule may cause perihepatitis (Fitz-Hugh-Curtis syndrome). This results in right hypochondrial pain and tenderness which may be mistaken for cholecystitis. A high index of suspicion is required as the accompanying salpingitis may be covert. Infertility due to bilateral tubal obstruction is a frequent complication of untreated and recurrent chlamydial salpingitis, and there is a risk of ectopic pregnancy in women due to incomplete occlusion of the tubes resulting from fibrosis.

In children
Chlamydial infection of the birth canal leads to neonatal conjunctivitis (Fig. 24) in 50% of those exposed. Symptoms that develop about 1 week after birth are usually mild and self-limiting. Aspiration of infected material results in pneumonia (Fig. 23) in about 10% of neonates exposed. This usually occurs at 2–3 months of age, and whilst not life-threatening, may result in significant lung damage. It is also postulated that the neonatal vagina may become infected at birth and that this infection may not be detected for several years. The possibility of sexual abuse in such cases however, should always be carefully considered. ➡

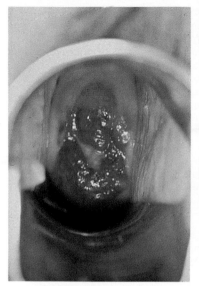

Fig. 22 Chlamydial cervicitis.

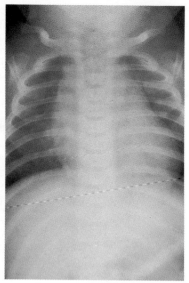

Fig. 23 Chlamydial pneumonitis in an infant.

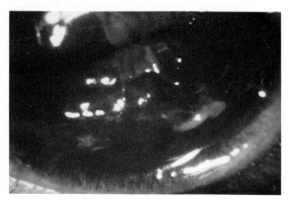

Fig. 24 Chlamydial conjunctivitis in a neonate.

NGU in men implies that the diagnosis is one of exclusion, and essentially this is the case. NGU is diagnosed if a Gram-stained smear from the urethra reveals numerous pus cells but no Gram-negative diplococci, and gonococcal culture is negative. The precise number of pus cells regarded as significant varies among centres, but the authors regard 5–10 pus cells per high-power field as indicative of urethritis. If facilities allow, the diagnosis may be supported by detection of chlamydiae.

No such clear-cut guidelines for the diagnosis of NSGI exist in women. The decision to treat is often based on epidemiological grounds supported by screening for chlamydial infection.

Chlamydial infection
Chlamydial DNA may be detected by PCR or LCR in endocervical material obtained with a cotton wool-tipped applicator stick or in a first-voided sample of urine. Alternatively, chlamydial isolation (Figs 25 & 26) may be attempted in tissue-cell cultures for which clinical specimens should be placed in a special transport medium such as 2SP. Chlamydial antigens may also be detected by enzyme immunoassay or immunofluorescence.

Doxycycline or Deteclo, both given orally for 7 d are usually effective; azithromycin given as a single oral dose or a 7-day course of ofloxacin are reasonable alternatives. With the possible exception of azithromycin, however, these drugs are contraindicated in pregnancy, when erythromycin may be used instead. Partner notification is essential. Epidemiological treatment of female partners of men with NGU is widely favoured.

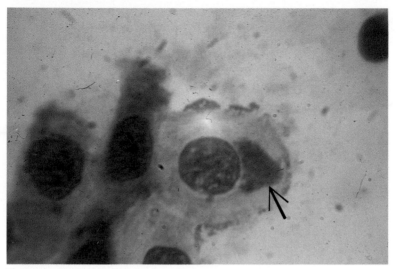

Fig. 25 Inclusion bodies of chlamydiae (Giemsa stain).

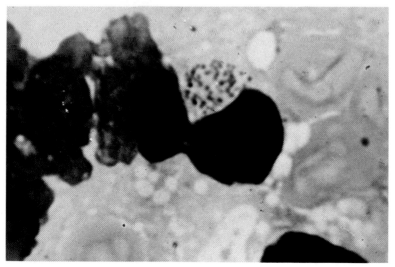

Fig. 26 Reticulate bodies of chlamydiae.

8 / Reiter's syndrome

Definition

In 1916 the triad of urethritis, arthritis and conjunctivitis was described by Hans Reiter. The major component of Reiter's syndrome (RS) is the arthropathy, and the other features are not invariably present. The syndrome may follow either gastrointestinal infection (due to salmonella, shigella, yersinia or campylobacter) or genitourinary infection (due to chlamydiae and possibly other agents). The acronyms EARA (enterically acquired reactive arthritis) and SARA (sexually acquired reactive arthritis) have also been proposed for these two forms.

Genetic factors

The histocompatibility antigen HLA B27 is present in up to 80% of patients with RS. The syndrome overlaps with ankylosing spondylitis that is also associated with HLA B27. The male:female ratio is approximately 50:1.

Clinical features

The postvenereal form is more commonly seen in the UK, and follows NGU in approximately 1% of cases. The onset is acute, occurring 2–3 weeks postinfection. Only a few joints are affected, classically knees and ankles (Fig. 27), although other large joints may be involved. Joint rupture may occur occasionally.

Sacroiliitis (Fig. 28) is common whereas inflammation of the small joints of hands and feet is not. Urethritis is indistinguishable from other forms of NGU. Conjunctivitis (Figs 29 & 30) is present in one-third of cases and is bilateral.

Other common features include tenosynovitis (especially of the Achilles' tendon), plantar fasciitis, circinate balanitis and keratoderma blennorrhagica. Less common are uveitis, lesions of the oral mucosa, carditis, glomerulonephritis and thrombophlebitis (Figs 31–36, pp. 28 & 30). ➤

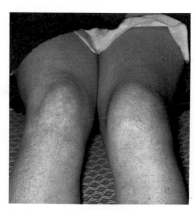

Fig. 27 Arthritis of knee joint.

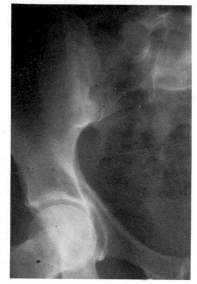

Fig. 28 Sacroiliitis.

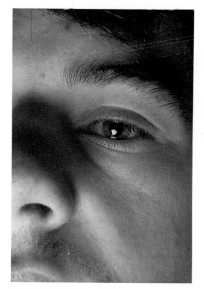

Fig. 29 Mild conjunctivitis.

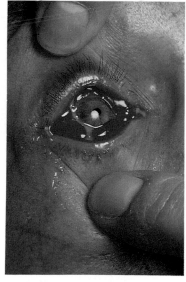

Fig. 30 Severe conjunctivitis.

Differential diagnosis

Gonococcal arthritis must be excluded by collection of appropriate specimens for gonococcal culture. It should be noted however that as gonococcal and chlamydial infections frequently co-exist, 5% of patients with RS initially present with gonorrhoea. Rheumatoid arthritis is usually excluded by the pattern of joint involvement, the presence of urethritis, and the absence of IgM rheumatoid factor. Ankylosing spondylitis and other seronegative arthropathies may be more difficult to exclude, but the presence of urethritis and acute onset of symptoms should be diagnostic.

Diagnosis

There is no diagnostic test for RS and the diagnosis is made on clinical grounds alone. The ESR is usually raised and HLA B27 is often present. ➡

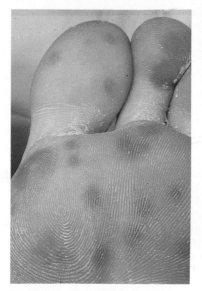

Fig. 31 Keratoderma blenorrhagica.

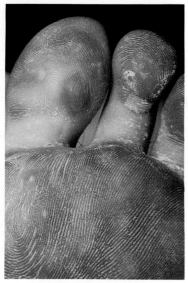

Fig. 32 Keratoderma blenorrhagica.

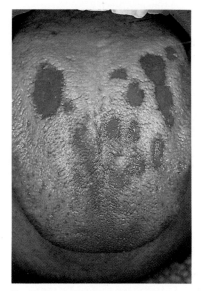

Fig. 33 Mucosal lesions of the tongue.

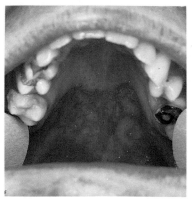

Fig. 34 Petechial lesions of the palate.

Treatment	Urethritis is managed conventionally with a tetracycline and usually clears promptly. As the arthropathy usually resolves within 3–6 months, symptomatic therapy alone is indicated. Aspirin may be sufficient to control joint inflammation, but commonly a more powerful anti-inflammatory drug such as naproxen or indomethacin is required. Acutely inflamed joints should be rested and physiotherapy instituted to prevent muscle wasting. Where a large effusion has accumulated in a joint, aspiration of fluid followed by instillation of methylprednisolone or indomethacin will give considerable relief.
	Conjunctivitis may be treated with saline lavage or betamethasone eye drops. Uveitis should be managed in conjunction with an ophthalmologist.
	Circinate balanitis (Figs 37 & 38) is treated with hydrocortisone cream.
	Keratoderma is difficult to treat but is self-limiting.
Prognosis	The majority of cases resolve within 3–6 months. Recurrences, however, are common. In some patients the arthropathy evolves to a chronic condition indistinguishable from ankylosing spondylitis.

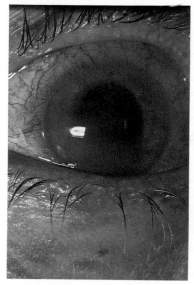

Fig. 35 Anterior uveitis.

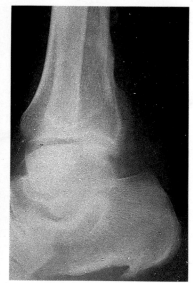

Fig. 36 Plantar spur.

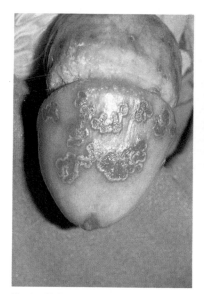

Fig. 37 Circinate balanitis.

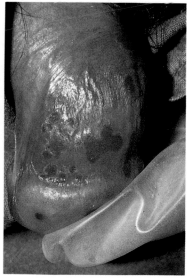

Fig. 38 Circinate balanitis.

9 / Gonorrhoea

Aetiology

Gonorrhoea is caused by the bacterium *Neisseria gonorrhoeae* (commonly referred to as the gonococcus) that infects mucosal surfaces of the genitourinary tract, rectum and pharynx.

Epidemiology

Gonorrhoea is transmitted almost exclusively by sexual contact. In the UK and USA it is one of the most prevalent infections after the childhood exanthemata. Incidence rates fell after the Second World War with the advent of antibiotics, then rose through the 1960s. The incidence has been falling since the mid-1970s. Rectal gonorrhoea in the male (reflecting homosexual contact) has fallen substantially in recent years as a result of changing sexual behaviour in the face of the epidemic of HIV infection. β-lactamase-producing strains of the organism are prevalent in South East Asia and in West Africa.

Clinical features

In males
Urethral infection is symptomatic in 90% of cases (Fig. 39). A purulent or mucopurulent discharge and/or dysuria develops after a prepatent period of 3–5 d (range 2–14 d). Complications are relatively rare, as patients tend to seek medical advice before these develop. Infection may spread to involve parafrenal (Tyson's) glands (Fig. 40), the epididymis, prostate, glans penis and median raphe (Fig. 41). Late complications such as urethral stricture are now extremely rare.

   Unilateral epididymo-orchitis (Fig. 42) is the most common complication, and prompt diagnosis and treatment is essential to prevent abscess formation. Disseminated gonococcal infection (DGI) is rare.

Pharyngeal infection as a result of orogenital contact rarely produces symptoms.

Rectal infection is also usually symptomless, although a few patients may complain of anal discharge, pain and tenesmus. Proctoscopy may reveal no clinical features of proctitis. ►

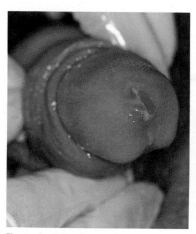

Fig. 39 Gonococcal urethritis.

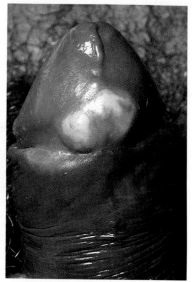

Fig. 40 Gonococcal infection of the parafrenal (Tyson's) glands.

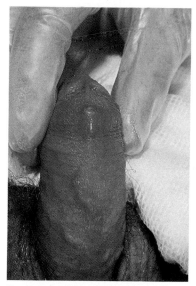

Fig. 41 Gonococal infection of the median raphe.

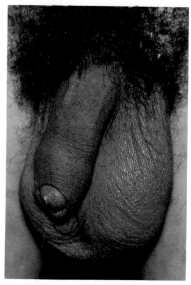

Fig. 42 Gonococcal epididymo-orchitis.

In adult females

Genital infection in the female is symptomless in over 70% of cases. The cervix (Fig. 43) is involved in 85–90% of cases, but the resultant discharge is profuse enough to be recognised in only 10%. Urethral infection (65–70%) is usually symptomless although there may be occasional dysuria and urinary frequency. Anorectal infection (30–50%) is almost invariably symptomless. The vagina is not infected. Pharyngeal infection as a result of fellatio is usually asymptomatic.

Complications: involvement of the greater vestibular (Bartholin's) gland may result in abscess formation. Ascending infection from the cervix resulting in gonococcal salpingitis occurs in 10% of cases. The presentation is usually acute with lower abdominal pain and fever. Clinical signs include pyrexia, lower abdominal tenderness, guarding, adnexal swelling and pain on cervical excitation during bimanual examination; there is a raised white cell count and ESR. Irreversible tubal damage may occur within 72 h and long-term sequelae include ectopic (tubal) pregnancy, and infertility if infection is bilateral. Inflammation of the liver capsule (perihepatitis) following spillage of infected tubal secretion into the peritoneum is a rare complication.

Disseminated gonococcal infection (Figs 44 & 45): haematogenous dissemination occurs in less than 1% of cases. Most patients with DGI have no genitourinary symptoms; the syndrome is more common in women. The main features are pyrexia, a vasculitic rash and polyarthritis; in some individuals, there is a monoarthritis (Fig. 46). Gonococcal culture from joint aspirate and blood is frequently negative, and the diagnosis is made from material obtained from the genital tract. ➤

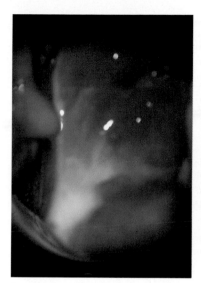

Fig. 43 Gonococcal cervicitis.

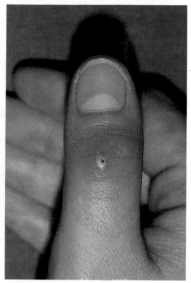

Fig. 44 Papulopustule of disseminated gonococcal infection.

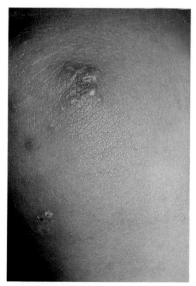

Fig. 45 Papulopustule of disseminated gonococcal infection.

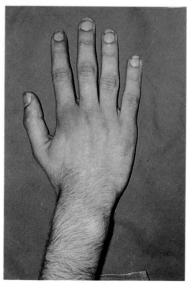

Fig. 46 Gonococcal arthritis.

In children
Ophthalmia neonatorum (Fig. 47): gonococcal cervicitis in pregnancy may lead to infection of the neonatal conjunctivae during birth. A purulent discharge usually develops within 48 h. If treatment is delayed, corneal scarring may result.

Vulvovaginitis (Fig. 48): the soft stratified squamous epithelium of prepubertal girls is susceptible to gonococcal infection. Vaginal discharge and vulval erythema are therefore more common than in adult women. Historically, the mode of acquisition has been considered to be accidental contamination, but this view has fallen into disfavour with the suspicion that up to 95% of cases may represent sexual abuse.

Diagnosis

In men
A Gram-stained smear of urethral exudate (Fig. 49) should be examined microscopically for Gram-negative diplococci, although every case should be confirmed by culture. As microscopy may be negative, material for culture should always be sent in a suitable transport medium such as Amies or Stuart's. Gonococci are cultured on a selective medium such as MNYC in a CO_2-enriched atmosphere, with identification of suspected colonies by oxidase reaction, sugar utilisation tests, coagglutination and immunofluorescence (Figs 50 & 51, p. 38). ▶

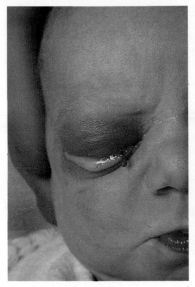

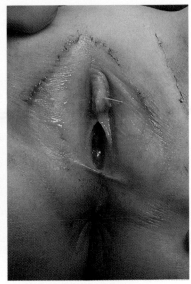

Fig. 47 Gonococcal ophthalmia neonatorum.

Fig. 48 Gonococcal vulvovaginitis.

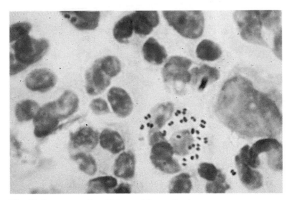

Fig. 49 Gram-negative diplococci in urethral smear.

Diagnosis

When oral or anal intercourse is suspected, material for culture should be taken from the pharynx and rectum on two occasions as infection of these sites is more difficult to diagnose.

In females
Microscopy of cervical material will be positive in less than 50% of cases. As the urethra and rectum are frequently colonised by the gonococcus (and may be the only affected sites) material for culture should be obtained from these sites in addition to the cervix. If the initial tests are negative, culture should be repeated at least once before gonococcal infection is excluded. A high vaginal swab will fail to diagnose 50% of infections.

Treatment

Single-dose therapy is adequate for uncomplicated genital infection in either sex. The choice of antimicrobial agent will depend on a knowledge of the antimicrobial sensitivities of the gonococcal strains prevalent in the area where the infection has been acquired. For example, in western Europe, amoxycillin given with probenecid to delay renal excretion is satisfactory for locally acquired infections. When gonorrhoea has been acquired in parts of the world where gonococcal strains with plasmid – or chromosomally mediated resistance to penicillin and other antimicrobial agents are common, cefotaxime, ceftriaxone or ofloxacin are better first-line treatments. More prolonged courses of therapy are needed for pharyngeal gonorrhoea and for complicated infection.

Co-infection with chlamydiae is present in 40% of heterosexual patients, and it is thus common practice to prescribe a course of tetracycline or erythromycin to be taken after completion of therapy for gonococcal infection. Contact tracing is essential.

At least one follow-up test should be performed at least 48–72 h after completion of therapy and in women this should include rectal sampling.

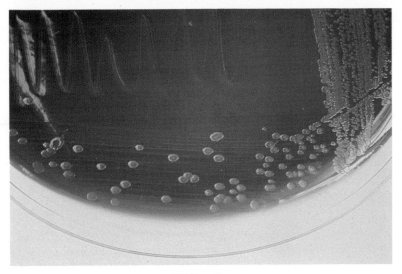

Fig. 50 Colonies of *N. gonorrhoeae* on MNYC medium.

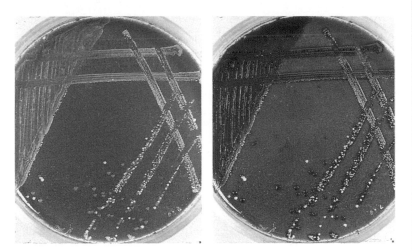

Fig. 51 Positive oxidase reaction with Neisseriae (white colonies are *S. epidermidis.*)

10 / Genital warts

Aetiology

Caused by the DNA-containing human papilloma virus (HPV). There are at least 80 different types that can be identified by DNA-DNA hybridisation methods. Genital warts are most commonly caused by types 6b and 11, but types 16 and 18 are sometimes found either singly or with the former types.

Epidemiology

The incidence of genital warts in the UK has been increasing over the past 20 years. Most individuals have acquired the virus through sexual contact, but although their presence may indicate sexual abuse, in children these warts may be acquired non-sexually. Laryngeal papillomata in children may result from infection as the child passes down the birth canal of an infected mother. Some infected individuals have subclinical lesions that can only be identified by colposcopy; they may represent a reservoir of infection in the community. One-third of patients with genital warts have a concurrent sexually transmitted infection. There is an association between certain HPV types (16, 18 – high risk; 31, 33, 35, 39, 45, 56 – intermediate risk) and premalignant and malignant disease of the genital tract. As healthy individuals can harbour these types, co-factors are probably important in carcinogenesis.

Clinical features

The prepatent period is very variable and difficult to define; warts may develop up to 2 years from contact with an infected person.

In males
Hyperplastic condylomata acuminata are found in the coronal sulcus, on the inner aspect of the prepuce (Fig. 52), at the urethral meatus (Fig. 53), in the perianal region (Fig. 54) and within the anal canal (Fig. 55). Sessile and plane warts may be found on the shaft of the penis. ➡

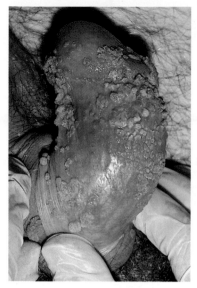

Fig. 52 Subpreputial warts.

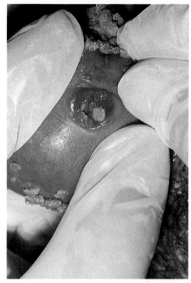

Fig. 53 Intrameatal warts.

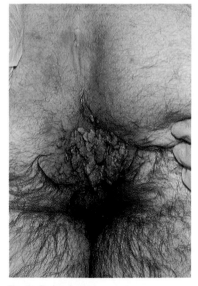

Fig. 54 Perianal warts.

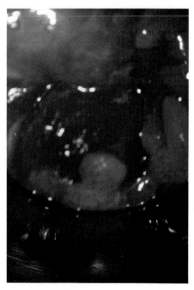

Fig. 55 Intra-anal warts.

In females

In women, condylomata acuminata are found at the introitus, on the labia minora and majora (Fig. 56), perineum, vagina, perianal region, urethra and cervix (Fig. 57). Although the cervix may appear normal macroscopically, by colposcopy, after the application of 5% acetic acid, slightly raised aceto-white areas may be seen in some women with HPV infection of that site (Fig. 58).

Dysplastic-like changes are found in cervical biopsies from up to 50% of women with genital warts. Spontaneous regression of lower grade HPV-associated cervical intra-epithelial neoplasia (CIN) is well recognised, but higher grades of HPV CIN may progress to carcinoma in situ or to invasive disease. Rarely, in both sexes, intra-oral condylomata occur.

In prepubertal children, condylomata may be found at the introitus, perineum and in the perianal region (Fig. 59).

Diagnosis

The diagnosis is clinical. Conditions that require differentiation include penile papillae, molluscum contagiosum, condylomata lata, and early squamous cell carcinoma.

Treatment

In the absence of specific antiviral therapy, treatment is aimed at controlling growth of the warts and reducing the risk of sepsis. Podophyllin resin suspended in liquid paraffin or ethanol, or, perhaps better, podophyllotoxin, should be applied topically at regular intervals until the lesions regress. Its use on the cervix, vagina or within the anal canal should be avoided, and as the drug can be absorbed systemically it should not be used in pregnancy. Cryotherapy, electrocautery or diathermy, and scissor excision are also used in treatment. The topical application of the immunomodulating drug imiquimod may be a helpful adjuvant to treatment.

Individuals should be screened for other STIs. Sexual contacts should be examined.

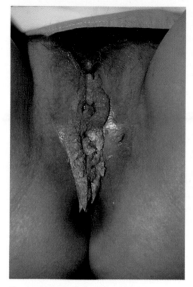

Fig. 56 Vulval warts.

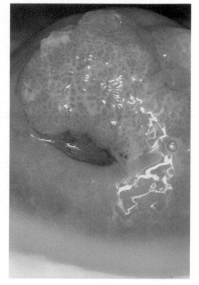

Fig. 57 Cervical condyloma.

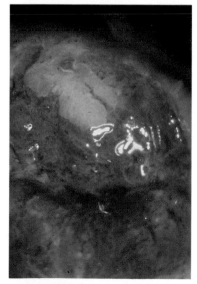

Fig. 58 Aceto-white areas of the cervix with HPV infection.

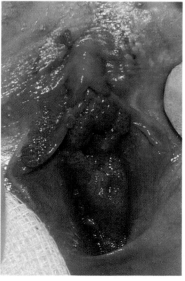

Fig. 59 Prepubertal introital warts.

11 / Genital herpes

Aetiology

There are two types of the DNA-containing herpes simplex virus (HSV) – types 1 and 2.

Pathogenesis

At the site of entry into the body through the skin or mucosae there is multiplication of virus with infection of nerve endings. Nucleocapsid is transported via the axon to the dorsal root ganglia where further multiplication occurs. Infectious virions then migrate centrifugally to the surface. After resolution of the primary infection, latency is established. Reactivation may occur with or without clinical disease.

Epidemiology

Over the past 15 years the prevalence of genital herpes in developed countries has increased. Although lesions at this site are associated classically with HSV-2, up to 50% of isolates are HSV-1. Symptomless excretion is probably important in maintaining the infection in the community. A previous HSV-1 infection may protect against acquisition of a clinically apparent HSV-2 infection.

Clinical features

Primary infections: genital lesions are accompanied by systemic symptoms – fever, headache, malaise and myalgia. Painful or itchy lesions develop with dysuria and sometimes a urethral or vaginal discharge. Multiple papules, vesicles or pustules that ulcerate appear on the genitalia (Figs 60, 61 & 62). After a variable period, crusting and healing occurs but new lesions may form. There is inguinal lymphadenitis. Lesions usually heal within 3–4 weeks. Extragenital lesions (Fig. 63), and sacral radiculitis may occur. Proctitis may result from anal intercourse (Fig. 64). HSV-1 primary infections tend to be less severe than those associated with HSV-2. ➡

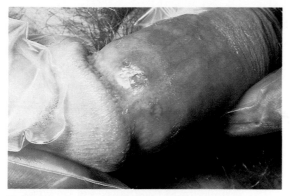

Fig. 60 Herpetic ulcer on the penis.

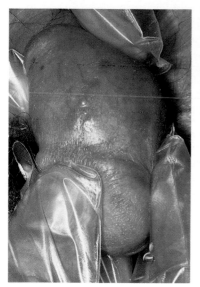

Fig. 61 Herpetic vesicle on the penis.

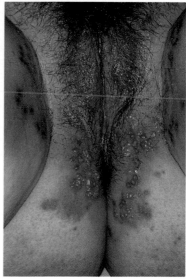

Fig. 62 Herpetic ulceration of the vulva.

**Clinical features
(contd)**

Initial infections: in patients with non-primary initial infections (i.e. persons who have clinical or serological evidence of prior HSV infection) the disease is milder than in those suffering primary infections.

Recurrent infections: the lesions of recurrent herpes resemble those of the initial episode but are localised to the genitalia, are of lesser extent, heal more quickly and are not associated with systemic features. There may be prodromal symptoms, e.g. tingling in the area. There is individual variation in the frequency of recurrences, but they are more likely in persons with HSV-2 infections. Symptomless recurrences are well documented.

Diagnosis

Diagnosis is by viral isolation in tissue culture, or antigen detection in material from lesions. Serology may be useful in primary infections.

Treatment

Acyclovir, valaciclovir or famciclovir given orally are invaluable in the treatment of primary and initial herpes; they may be used in recurrences but the effects are not so obvious. If given during the prodrome (if any) or within 24 h of the development of lesions, they may shorten the duration of a recurrence. In the case of individuals with frequent recurrences, say more than eight per year, or in immunocompromised patients, suppressive treatment with these drugs can be helpful. Drug resistance is rare.

Genital herpes in pregnancy
Primary HSV-2 infection during pregnancy, particularly during the third trimester, may be associated with prematurity and growth retardation. Infection during parturition is associated with high neonatal mortality. This can be prevented by delivery by Caesarean section before membrane rupture.
   The risk of neonatal herpes is much lower in women with recurrent disease.

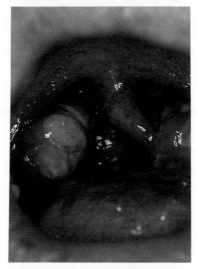

Fig. 63 Herpetic ulceration of the tonsils.

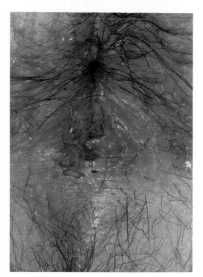

Fig. 64 Perianal herpes in a homosexual man.

12 / Molluscum contagiosum

Aetiology	Caused by a virus of the DNA-containing poxvirus group.
Epidemiology	Over the past decade the incidence in the UK has been increasing. The virus is transmitted by personal contact, including sexual, or by fomites.
Clinical features	After a prepatent period of 15–50 d, pearly, raised, firm, hemispherical papules about 2–5 mm in diameter and with an umbilicated centre appear either singly or in groups on the affected area (Figs 65). Although they may persist for many months, spontaneous regression usually occurs. In immunocompromised patients, including those with HIV infection, lesions can be extensive and persistent (Fig. 66).
Diagnosis	This is clinical, but can be confirmed by electron microscopy of material from the core.
Treatment	Piercing with a sharpened orange stick that has been dipped in tincture of iodine, cryotherapy, or electrocautery are effective. Sexual partners should be examined also. Following the immune restoration resulting from highly active antiretroviral therapy in HIV–infected individuals, lesions often regress spontaneously (Fig. 67).

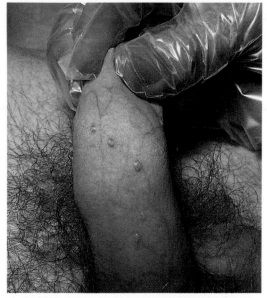

Fig. 65 Molluscum contagiosum of the shaft of the penis.

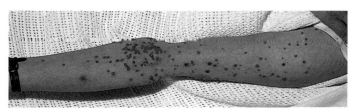

Fig. 66 Widespread molluscum contagiosum in an HIV-infected woman.

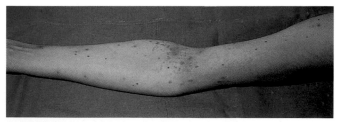

Fig. 67 Regression of lesions after initiation of antiretroviral therapy in the same patient.

13 / Hepatitis A

Aetiology	Caused by the RNA-containing hepatitis A virus (HAV).
Epidemiology	Very common infection in childhood in developing countries. Seroprevalence rates in industrialised counties have been falling over the past 3 decades. Faecal-oral transmission via person-to-person contact within households is the predominant mode of spread of HAV. Sporadic outbreaks of infection amongst homosexual men in whom transmission may be by oral-anal sex, digital anal intercourse, or penoinsertive anal intercourse. HAV is excreted in the faeces for up to 2 weeks before onset of illness and for about 1 week thereafter.
Clinical features	Symptomless and anicteric infections are common. Prepatent period of acute hepatitis A is 15–50 d. Prodromal features include fever, malaise, anorexia, nausea and vomiting, and precede the appearance of dark urine and the development of jaundice (if it occurs). Sometimes there is mild pruritus.
Diagnosis	This rests with the detection of specific IgM to HAV in the serum during the acute phase of the illness (Fig. 68).
Treatment	This is symptomatic.
Prevention	Vaccination should be offered to those at risk, including men who have sex with men.

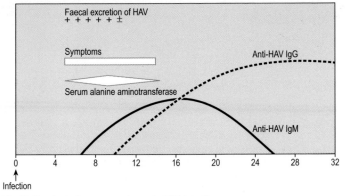

Fig. 68 Serological responses in acute HAV infection.

Aetiology	Caused by the DNA-containing hepatitis B virus (Fig. 69).
Epidemiology	Endemic in certain geographical areas where it may have been acquired perinatally. In western countries, it is spread sexually, particularly by homosexual anal intercourse, or parenterally as, for example, in i.v. drug misusers. Sex industry workers may be at increased risk of infection. Individuals whose serum contains e antigen are the most infectious.
Clinical features	Symptomless acute infections are common. Some persons develop acute icteric hepatitis (Fig. 70) after a prepatent period of 30–130 d. In a small proportion of patients, chronicity develops. Many of these individuals are well, without biochemical abnormalities of liver function. In others, chronic persistent or active hepatitis, cirrhosis or hepatocellular carcinoma may develop. Seroconversion from e antigenaemia to anti-e may occur eventually. In chronic hepatitis B, although anti-HBc IgG is detected, anti-HBc IgM is not found.
Treatment	That of acute illness is symptomatic. Interferon-alpha can be helpful in the treatment of patients with chronic hepatitis B, as may antiviral agents such as lamivudine given in combination with either interferon or another nucleoside analogue.
Prevention	Vaccine should be offered to those at risk.

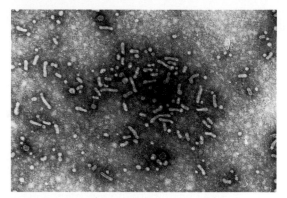

Fig. 69 Hepatitis B virus particles.

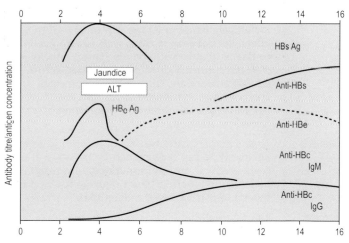

Fig. 70 Serological responses in acute hepatitis B virus infection.

15 / Hepatitis C

Aetiology | Caused by the RNA-containing hepatitis C virus (HCV).

Epidemiology | Blood-borne viral infection that is now most frequently transmitted through sharing contaminated equipment by i.v. drug users (Fig. 71). HCV can also be transmitted transplacentally, particularly when the maternal viral load is high. Sexual transmission occurs, but the risk of acquisition of HCV from an infected partner is low. Needle stick injury from an infected individual also carries a risk of infection.

Clinical features | Acute infection is usually symptomless; only a few individuals become icteric. Up to 85% of HCV infections become chronic with histological evidence of chronic hepatitis. These individuals may have normal or minimally raised serum aminotransferases. Cirrhosis is a common complication and the development of hepatocellular carcinoma in the setting of cirrhosis is well-recognised.

Diagnosis | This is made by the testing of serum for antibody against HCV, but the test can be negative in very early infection and in immunocompromised patients. Polymerase chain reaction for viral RNA is helpful in confirming the diagnosis.

Treatment | Interferon-alpha with or without ribavirin is helpful in some cases.

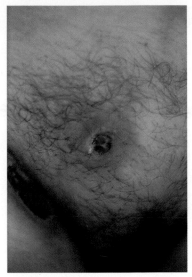

Fig. 71 Most new infections with HCV are acquired through sharing contaminated syringes and needles.

Epstein–Barr virus

Clinical features

The Epstein–Barr (EBV) virus is a herpes virus present in saliva and can be transmitted by kissing. Its presence in cervical epithelial cells suggests that it can be acquired also by sexual intercourse.

The virus is usually acquired in childhood when infection is inapparent. When infection is delayed until adolescence or early adulthood, 50% of individuals develop the clinical features of infectious mononucleosis: malaise, fever, sore throat with a pharyngeal exudate (Fig. 72), a maculopapular skin rash, generalised lymphnode enlargement, splenomegaly, sometimes mild icterus, and features of meningism. These features usually resolve within about 2 weeks, but a protracted illness may occur.

Diagnosis

The diagnosis is suggested by finding an absolute lymphocytosis with many atypical or pleomorphic cells (Fig. 73); a finding of heterophil antibodies detected by the monospot slide test confirms the diagnosis.

Cytomegalovirus

Cytomegalovirus (CMV) can be transmitted hetero- and homosexually, vertically to the fetus, by breast-milk, or possibly by kissing.

Clinical features

Primary infection is usually symptomless, but a mononucleosis-like illness may develop; in this case however, the monospot test is negative. In immunodeficient individuals, e.g. people with acquired immune deficiency syndrome (AIDS), retinitis, pneumonia or colitis may occur. Congenital infection may produce no obvious effects, mental retardation, or be associated with the classical features of microcephaly, hepatosplenomegaly, chorioretinitis, uveitis or purpura.

Diagnosis

Diagnosis is by culture of the virus or from the urine or pharyngeal secretions or by serology.

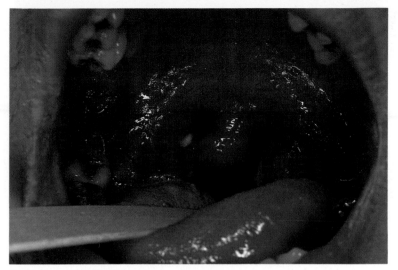

Fig. 72 Pharyngitis of EBV.

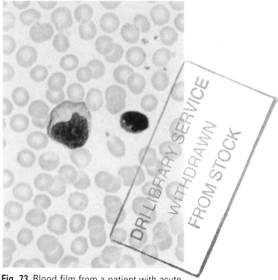

Fig. 73 Blood film from a patient with acute mononucleosis.

17 / Human immunodeficiency virus infection

Aetiology

The human immunodeficiency viruses (HIV) are RNA-containing retroviruses (Fig. 74) that attack cells that bear the CD4 receptor lymphocytes: macrophages, Langerhans' cells and microglia, and interfere with cellular immunity. Other receptors are also important for viral entry into these cells.

Natural history of HIV infection

Within a few days of infection, the virus becomes detectable in the blood, and after peaking, the concentration falls to become fairly constant at a level that varies from individual to individual (so called 'set-point'). Patients with a high viral load (as measured by the concentration of viral RNA in the plasma) develop symptomatic disease much more quickly than those with a low viral load. Estimation of the plasma viral load then can be helpful in planning treatment (see below). Shortly after infection, the CD4$^+$ cell count in the peripheral blood falls, but as the plasma viraemia decreases, it rises only to fall thereafter at a rate that shows much inter-person variation (Fig. 75). When the CD4$^+$ cell count falls below 200/mm^3, the individual is at risk of opportunistic infection. Untreated, 50% of HIV-infected individuals developed an AIDS-defining illness within 10 years of infection.

Epidemiology

The viruses that are present in blood, semen, and cervico-vaginal secretions, can be transmitted sexually – both homo- and heterosexually – by transfusion of contaminated blood or by contaminated syringes and needles. Concurrent STIs may facilitate sexual transmission of HIV. They can also be transmitted to the fetus from an infected mother.

The prevalence of HIV-1 infection varies geographically but is high in some areas (e.g. central Africa). In industrialised countries, the incidence of infection amongst men who have sex with other men may be decreasing, although it continues to rise amongst younger homosexual men.

HIV-2 is endemic in west Africa.

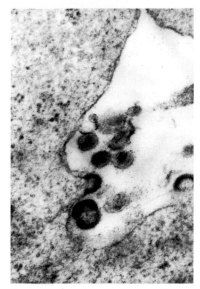

Fig. 74 Electron photomicrograph of HIV-1.

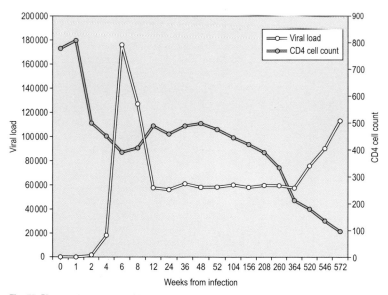

Fig. 75 Plasma viral load and CD4⁺ cell count in peripheral blood of an untreated HIV-infected individual.

Most HIV-infected persons are symptomless. Shortly before seroconversion, a proportion develop a mononucleosis-like illness with abrupt onset of fever, headache, arthralgia, myalgia, diarrhoea, a maculopapular skin rash (Figs 76 & 77), generalised lymphadenopathy, aphthous ulceration of the mouth or candidiasis (Fig. 78). Meningoencephalitis may occur. These features usually resolve within about 2 weeks. Persistent generalised lymphadenopathy is common and affects at least two non-contiguous sites. The enlargement is usually symptomless. The nodes are firm, mobile, discrete and non-tender. Histologically there is usually reactive hyperplasia; involution may herald onset of secondary infections. In an HIV-seropositive individual, biopsy in not indicated unless there is doubt about the diagnosis, and lymphoma or infections such as tuberculosis are considered. ➡

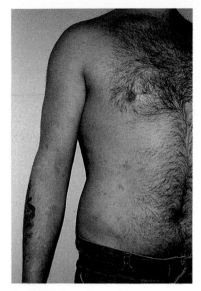

Fig. 76 Rash associated with seroconversion.

Fig. 77 Rash associated with seroconversion.

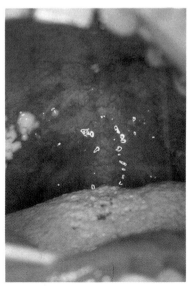

Fig. 78 Oral candidiasis associated with seroconversion.

Skin lesions are frequent. Few of these are specific for HIV, but they are often more extensive and recalcitrant to treatment than in immunocompetent individuals. Lesions include seborrhoeic dermatitis of the face, chest and upper arms (Fig. 79); folliculitis of the beard area (Fig. 80), chest, arms and thighs; mutiple molluscum contagiosum (p. 47); extensive tinea pedis and cruris; frequently recurring HSV infection; multiple dermatomal herpes zoster; recalcitrant anogenital warts; xeroderma. Purpura may be a feature of thrombocytopenia. Oral hairy leukoplakia affects the lateral borders of the tongue (Fig. 81); pseudomembranous or erythematous candidiasis, angular cheilitis, erosive gingivitis and aphthous ulceration are other oral manifestations (Fig. 82).

Additional features that herald the onset of serious disease include weight loss, febrile episodes, night sweats, persistent diarrhoea and lethargy. Features of dementia may also develop.

Some of the secondary infections and neoplasms that are indicative of cellular immunodeficiency are considered on pp. 63–69.

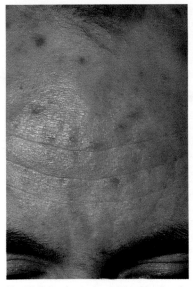

Fig. 79 Seborrhoeic dermatitis of forehead.

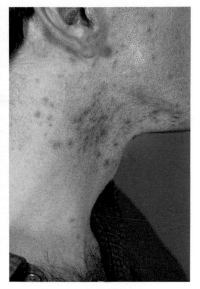

Fig. 80 Folliculitis of the beard area.

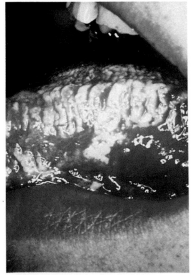

Fig. 81 Oral hairy leukoplakia.

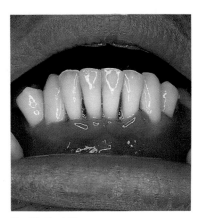

Fig. 82 Gingivitis.

Protozoal infections

Pneumocystis carinii is the most common opportunistic infection in AIDS. The pneumonia presents as increasing dyspnoea, non-productive cough and chest pain. In the early stages, there may be few signs; later, widespread coarse crepitations may be heard. Chest X-ray may be normal or show diffuse shadowing (Fig. 83). Diagnosis is by the detection of cysts in induced sputum, bronchoalveolar washings, or in biopsy material (Fig. 84). In ill patients, the usual treatment is with i.v. co-trimoxazole or pentamidine, both given with a glucocorticoid. Skin rashes with leucopenia or thrombocytopenia are common with co-trimoxazole. In less sick individuals, co-trimoxazole can be given orally; atovaquone is an alternative treatment. After resolution, prophylactic treatment with oral co-trimoxazole, dapsone or atovaquone, or with nebulised pentamidine is advised unless there is immune reconstitution by the use of antiviral drugs (pp. 73–75).

Toxoplasma gondii infestation can be disseminated or present as cerebral abscesses with focal features. Diagnosis is by serology and imaging procedures (Fig. 85). Findings in the latter are non-specific but allow a tentative diagnosis to be made. Treatment is with sulphamethoxazole and pyrimethamine. Prophylactic treatment is recommended after resolution of infection.

Cryptosporidium spp. affects the intestinal mucosa and causes severe diarrhoea. Diagnosis is by finding oocysts in faeces (Fig. 86) or biopsy material. Although there is no specific treatment, there is often resolution of infection when immune function improves after the initiation of highly active antiretroviral therapy (HAART).

Isospora belli is another cause of diarrhoea. Co-trimoxazole is the treatment of choice, but recurrence is common.

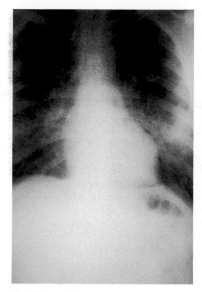

Fig. 83 *P. carinii* pneumonia.

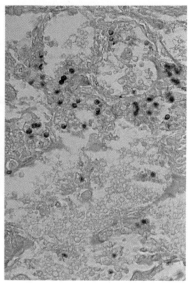

Fig. 84 *P. carinii* in a lung biopsy.

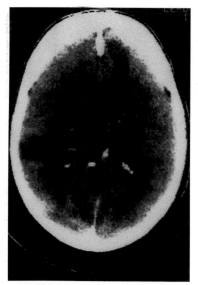

Fig. 85 CT scan of cerebral toxoplasmosis.

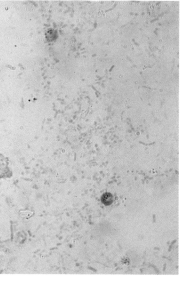

Fig. 86 Cryptosporidum oocysts in faeces.

Bacterial infections

Mycobacterium tuberculosis may cause pulmonary disease alone or can be disseminated. Treatment is with standard anti-tuberculous chemotherapy, although the emergence of multi-drug-resistant *M. tuberculosis* is now becoming a major problem. Atypical mycobacteria are associated with disseminated infection involving multiple organs. The intestinal tract may be severely affected. Diagnosis is by the detection of the bacteria in blood, sputum, faeces, or other bodily fluids or in biopsy material (Fig. 87). Treatment with a combination of clarithromycin, ethambutol and, possibly, rifabutin can be useful. Resolution may follow the initiation of HAART.

Streptococcus pneumoniae and *Haemophilus influenzae* are causes of pneumonia (Fig. 88). Diagnosis is by the detection of the bacteria in sputum or bronchoalveolar washings. Treatment is with an antibiotic to which the isolate is sensitive. As soon as possible after diagnosis of HIV infection, and particularly when the individual is severely immunocompromised, vaccination against both organisms should be offered.

Campylobacter spp. can cause diarrhoea. Bacteria may be difficult to find in the faeces and colonic biopsy may be necessary. Erythromycin or tetracyclines are used in treatment.

Shigella spp., especially *S. flexneri*, *Salmonella enteritidis* and *S. typhimurium* can cause diarrhoea and bacteraemia is common. Diagnosis is by culture of faeces and blood. Treatment is with an appropriate antibiotic, and, as recurrence is common, prophylaxis should be considered.

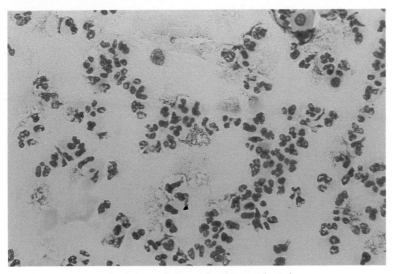

Fig. 87 Ziehl–Neelsen-stained smear of sputum showing mycobacteria.

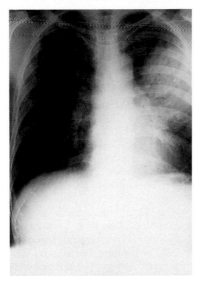

Fig. 88 Lobar pneumonia.

Fungal infections

Candida spp. Extensive superficial infection of mucosal surfaces is common. Oesophageal disease may cause dysphagia (Fig. 89). Chronic vulvovaginitis is often troublesome. Dissemination is rare, but cerebral abscesses can occur. Treatment is with oral fluconazole, ketoconazole or itraconazole and with topical antifungal preparations. Although recurrence is common in untreated patients, the use of HAART reduces the risk.

Cryptococcus neoformans is the commonest cause of meningitis in patients with AIDS. There may be few clinical features of meningitis. Diagnosis is by finding yeasts or antigen in the CSF. Intravenous amphotericin B, preferably liposomal, with or without 5-flucytosine, or oral fluconazole are used in treatment.

Viral infections

Cytomegalovirus (CMV) is very common, but isolation from clinical material does not necessarily indicate a pathogenic role in a disease process. Often disseminated, CMV can cause retinitis (Fig. 90), colitis and pneumonia. CMV can also cause painful anogenital and oesophageal ulceration. Ganciclovir and foscarnet are useful in treatment, as is cidofovir. Relapse is common but the risk is much reduced in patients receiving HAART.

Herpes simplex virus can cause extensive ulceration of the anogenital tract and facial region (Fig. 91). Aciclovir, valaciclovir and famciclovir are helpful in treatment and prophylaxis.

Herpes zoster (Fig. 92) is a common infection and is treated with aciclovir, valaciclovir or famciclovir.

JC virus is associated with progressive multifocal leucoencephalopathy, a cause of dementia. Diagnosis is by imaging, the detection of viral DNA in CSF, or biopsy. There is no well-established treatment, although cidofovir may be useful.

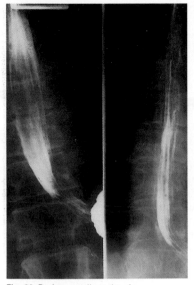

Fig. 89 Barium swallow showing oesophageal candidiasis.

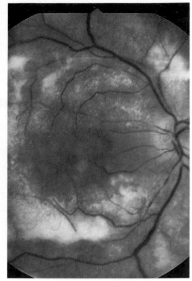

Fig. 90 CMV retinitis.

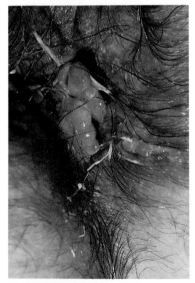

Fig. 91 Oedematous perianal skin tags in association with HSV.

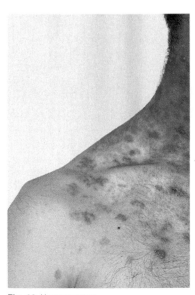

Fig. 92 Herpes zoster.

Neoplasms

Kaposi's sarcoma, a tumour of the endothelium, is associated with the human herpes virus 8 (HHV 8). The incidence of the tumour amongst homosexual men, the population group that was most commonly affected, has fallen over the past decade. The lesions are usually painless and non-pruritic, multiple, and affect any area of the body (Figs 93 & 94), including the head and neck. Mucosal involvement and visceral spread are common (Fig. 95). Localised lesions may not require treatment unless they are on the face or in the oral cavity, when they may respond to intralesional vincristine or radiotherapy.

Disseminated disease may require systemic therapy with cytotoxic drugs. Lesions often regress spontaneously after the initiation of HAART.

B-cell lymphomas commonly affect the gastrointestinal tract and brain. They are usually high grade but sometimes respond to chemotherapy, and in the case of cerebral lymphoma, to irradiation.

Squamous cell carcinomas of the anal canal, usually associated with HPV infection, may develop in HIV-infected individuals. Higher grade cervical intra-epithelial neoplasia is common in HIV-infected women who require regular colposcopic examination. Carcinoma of the tongue has also been reported.

HIV encephalopathy

Subcortical dementia may be a late feature of HIV infection, in the absence of other causes. Neuroimaging shows cortical atrophy (Fig. 96), sometimes with parenchymal lesions. Other causes of dementia must be excluded. Other neurological features include peripheral and autonomic neuropathy and vacuolar myelopathy; myositis may also be a feature. ➡

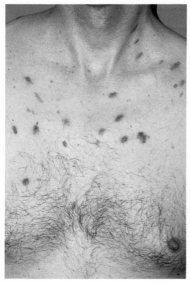

Fig. 93 Disseminated Kaposi's sarcoma.

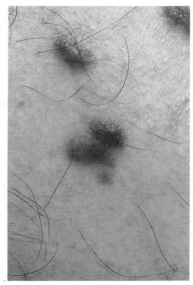

Fig. 94 Nodular lesion of Kaposi's sarcoma.

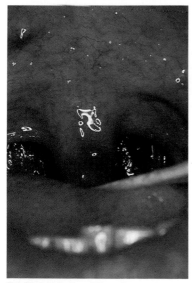

Fig. 95 Oral lesion of Kaposi's sarcoma.

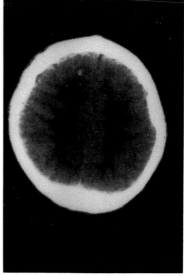

Fig. 96 CT scan showing cerebral atrophy.

Enzyme-linked immunosorbent assay (ELISA) methods for detecting antibodies against envelope proteins are used for screening; positive results are confirmed by another test, e.g. Western blot. These antibodies become detectable at a variable interval from infection that is unlikely to exceed 3 months. During acute HIV infection (seroconversion illness), the antibody test is usually negative but becomes positive within about 2 weeks of the onset of symptoms (Fig. 97). At this stage, the detection of viral RNA by a PCR is the investigation of choice. HIV core antigen can be detected in the peripheral blood early in infection, but becomes undetectable as antibody develops. Later, reappearance of antigen may be found to precede the development of serious disease. Where available, PCR for the detection of plasma RNA has almost replaced the antigen detection test.

At the time of diagnosis, in addition to taking a full medical and social history and undertaking a careful clinical examination, blood should be obtained for estimation of the $CD4^+$ cell count and the plasma concentration of viral RNA (viral load); unless the patient is symptomatic on account of HIV and the former test shows severe immunodeficiency, these tests should be repeated about 2–4 weeks later to obtain more precise data on which to base treatment decisions. Other baseline investigations that can be helpful in future management include:
1. Serological testing for previous infection with CMV, *Toxoplasma gondii*, hepatitis A, B and C viruses, syphilis
2. Chest X-ray
3. Tuberculin testing.

Untreated and symptomless patients are generally followed up at 3-monthly intervals at which time there is a physical examination, including measuring the weight, and the plasma viral load and $CD4^+$ cell count in the peripheral blood are estimated. Unexpected findings in these tests may necessitate more intensive surveillance. ➡

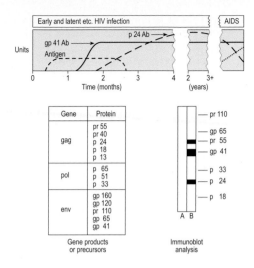

Gene	Protein
gag	pr 55 pr 40 p 24 p 18 p 13
pol	p 65 p 51 p 33
env	gp 160 gp 120 pr 110 gp 65 gp 41

Gene products
or precursors

Immunoblot
analysis

Fig. 97 Serological responses in HIV infection.

Treatment is aimed at long-term viral suppression and the restoration of immune function. Criteria for initiation of therapy vary, but treatment should be considered when the patient is symptomatic (possibly including those with primary infection), has a low or falling $CD4^+$ cell count in the peripheral blood, and a high viral load (>10 000 copies of viral RNA per mm^3). Although there are several therapeutic options for treatment-naïve individuals, at least three drugs should be used in combination.

The initial treatment regimen often comprises two nucleoside analogue reverse transcriptase inhibitors (for example, zidovudine and didanosine, zidovudine and lamivudine, stavudine and lamivudine, and lamivudine and didanosine) and either a non-nucleoside reverse transcriptase inhibitor (for example, nevirapine and efavirenz) or a protease inhibitor (for example, nelfinavir, indinavir, ritonavir and saquinavir).

With any regimen, patient adherence is essential to avoid the emergence of drug resistance and it is good to involve the individual in discussions about the choice of drugs. Treatment monitoring that includes clinical assessment for improvement or worsening of symptoms, estimation of plasma viral load, the $CD4^+$ cell count (Fig. 98), and haematological and biochemical tests to detect drug toxicity, should be undertaken at regular intervals, say every 3 months, after initiation of therapy. Side-effects from the nucleoside RT inhibitors include: nausea, diarrhoea, peripheral neuropathy (especially with zalcitabine and stavudine), anaemia (zidovudine), pancreatitis (didanosine) and myopathy (zidovudine). Skin rashes (Fig. 99), including erythema multiforme exudativum (Stevens–Johnson syndrome) may complicate treatment with nevirapine and efavirenz, and acute hypersensitivity reaction has been described with the nucleoside analogue abacavir. Lipodystrophy, hypertriglyceridaemia, hyperglycaemia, nephrolithiasis (indinavir) and circumoral and peripheral paraesthesiae (ritonavir), and peripheral neuropathy may be associated with the use of the protease inhibitors. ➡

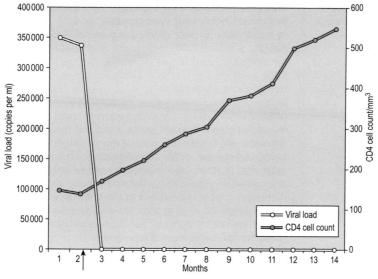

Fig. 98 Viral load and CD4⁺ cell response to successful antiretroviral therapy (combination treatment with zidovudine, didanosine and nevirapine, initiated at ↑).

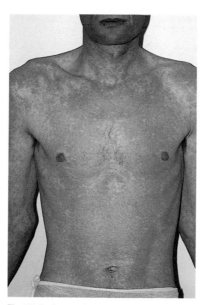

Fig. 99 Rash associated with nevirapine therapy.

Treatment failure, as is indicated by a symptomless individual becoming symptomatic, or a symptomatic patient developing an AIDS-defining illness, a falling $CD4^+$ cell count, and viral RNA becoming detectable again in the plasma (Fig. 100), may be the result of viral resistance, non-compliance, pharmacological failure (for example, enhanced drug metabolism or defective phosphorylation), poor drug potency, and malabsorption. The choice of a second treatment regimen must take account of the possibility of cross-resistance within the classes of drugs, their side-effects (that may influence patient adherence), and possible interactions between these agents. Although many individuals achieve long-term suppression of viral replication and sustained improvement in immune function, a substantial minority fail to achieve these goals.

Prevention

In the absence of an effective vaccine, control of infection depends on health education, e.g. encouraging the adoption of safer sexual practices and the avoidance of sharing non-sterile needles/syringes. The use of combination antiretroviral therapy in a pregnant woman and the administration of zidovudine to the new born infant reduces significantly the risk of neonatal infection. As maternal milk is an important source of neonatal infection, breastfeeding should be strongly discouraged. The use of antiretroviral drugs after significant exposure to HIV should be discussed. Injury is best avoided, however, by careful attention to detail when using or disposing of contaminated medical equipment (Fig. 101).

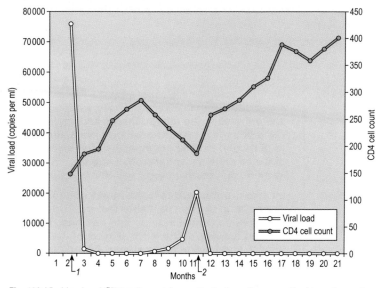

Fig. 100 Viral load and CD4 cell count in a patient whose therapy with zidovudine and lamivudine (initiated at ↑ 1) failed, but who subsequently responded to treatment with stavudine, didanosine and indinavir (initiated at ↑ 2).

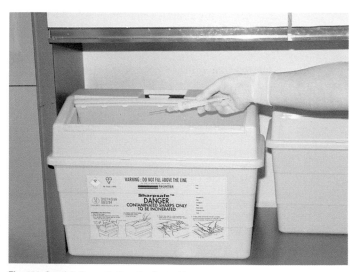

Fig. 101 Careful disposal of contaminated instruments.

18 / Genital candidiasis

Aetiology

Genital candidiasis is caused by species of yeasts, especially *Candida albicans*. These are found as saprophytes in the mouth, faeces and vagina. Conditions that favour transition from saprophyte to pathogen include pregnancy, tissue maceration, diabetes mellitus, antimicrobial agents, immunosuppressive drugs and HIV infection.

Clinical features

Intense pruritus vulvae is the most common symptom in the female. Other features include dyspareunia, vulval burning and swelling. There is marked redness of the inner aspects of the labia minora and vestibule sometimes extending to the labia majora, perineum and perianal skin. White plaques of variable size are found in the vagina, which may be reddened (Fig. 102). Primary cutaneous candidiasis affects the outer labia majora and genitocrural folds (Fig. 103), and presents as a weeping erythematous area with a scaly margin and small satellite pustules. In the male, there is soreness or itching of the penis with a subpreputial discharge. The glans and mucosal surface of the prepuce are inflamed with superfical erosions and preputial oedema (Fig. 104). A similar picture may result from hypersensitivity to candidal antigens and develop within 6–24 h of intercourse with an infected partner.

Diagnosis

Pseudohyphae in Gram-stained smears (Fig. 105), or culture on a glucose peptone agar (Sabouraud's).

Treatment

Antifungal imidazoles (e.g. clotrimazole) as cream or pessaries. Fluconazole or itraconazole, triazole antifungal agents, given as a single oral dose are highly effective alternative treatments. Women with frequent recurrences of candidiasis may benefit from suppressive treatment given around the anticipated time of recurrence, for example, pre-menstrually.

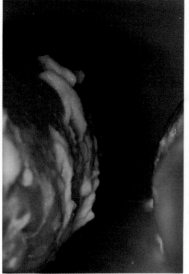

Fig. 102 Candidal vaginitis.

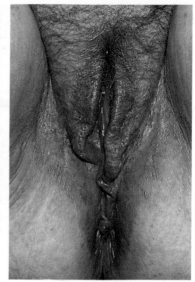

Fig. 103 Candidal vulvitis.

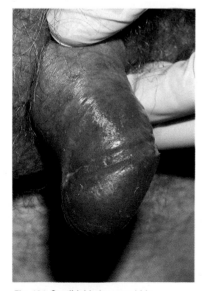

Fig. 104 Candidal balanoposthitis.

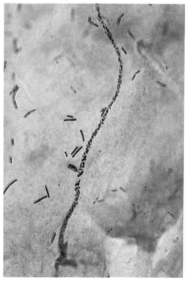

Fig. 105 Pseudohyphae of *Candida* species.

Aetiology

Although no single bacterium is responsible, *Gardnerella vaginalis* and anaerobes such as *Mobiluncus* spp., peptostreptococci and *Bacteroides* spp. (except *B. fragilis*) are associated with this clinical entity. The diamines putrescine and cadaverine and gamma-amino-n-butyric acid produced by the anaerobes are found in the vaginal discharge. There is no convincing evidence that the condition is sexually transmissible.

Clinical features

The patient complains of an increased vaginal discharge with a fishy odour that is most noticeable during and after sexual intercourse. Pruritus vulvae is not a feature. There is a homogeneous grey-white discharge that may coat the vaginal walls and pool in the posterior fornix. Although the mucosa may be mildly oedematous, vaginitis is not a feature. Bacterial vaginosis may be associated with infection following gynaecological surgery, low birth weight, and, possibly, miscarriage.

Diagnosis

Diagnosis is by recognition of the clinical features. The pH of infected vaginal secretions is higher than normal, generally > 5.0. A characteristic odour is produced on mixing a drop of vaginal secretion and KOH on a slide. Infection produces a positive 'sniff test'. 'Clue cells' can be seen in a saline mount of secretion (Fig. 106). In a Gram-stained smear (Fig. 107), there are few bacteria of the *Lactobacillus* morphotype, but increased numbers of small Gram-negative rods. Other forms of Gram-negative rods and Gram-positive cocci are also found.

Treatment

Metronidazole given as a single oral dose or intra-vaginal clindamycin cream are effective. Relapse, however, is common.

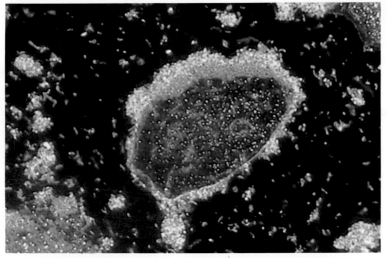

Fig. 106 Dark-field appearance of wet mount of vaginal material from bacterial vaginosis.

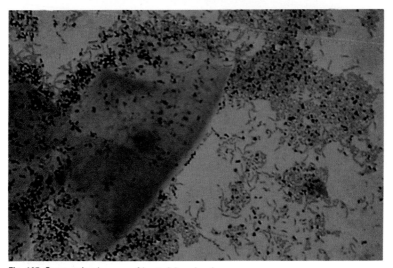

Fig. 107 Gram-stained smear of bacterial vaginosis.

Aetiology

Trichomonas vaginalis is a flagellated protozoon (Fig. 108) that invades the superficial epithelial cells of the vagina, urethra, glans penis, prostate and seminal vesicles.

Epidemiology

The organism is almost always sexually transmitted but, rarely, female neonates can be infected during delivery. In the UK incidence has been decreasing. Concurrent sexually transmitted infections are common.

Clinical features

In the female, the most common symptoms are vaginal discharge with an unpleasant odour, vulval soreness, dyspareunia and dysuria. Some women are symptomless. There is a variable degree of vaginitis and vulvitis (Fig. 109). The vaginal discharge is also variable; the classical frothy yellow discharge is found in less than one-third of infested women. Most infested men are symptomless, but urethritis and balanoposthitis may occur.

Diagnosis

Trichomonads may be found by direct microscopy or culture of vaginal exudate, or in the male, of urethral scrapings, prostatic fluid or centrifuged deposit of urine. The protozoon is sometimes found in Papanicolaou-stained cytology preparations. Specimens that cannot be examined immediately should be sent to the laboratory in a transport medium (e.g. Amies).

Treatment

Metronidazole is the treatment of choice. Although rare, resistance to this drug has been reported. Alcohol should be avoided during treatment with metronidazole. Regular partners should be examined and treated.

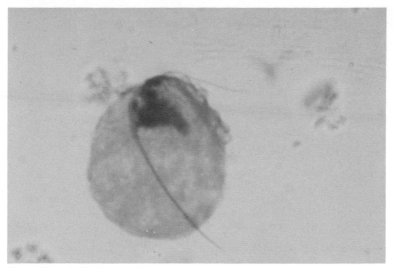

Fig. 108 *T. vaginalis* (Giemsa stain).

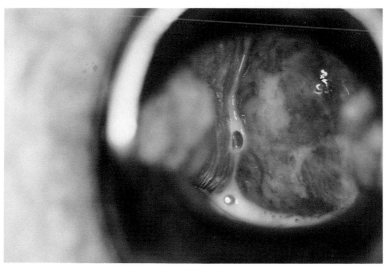

Fig. 109 Trichomonal vaginitis.

21 / Enteric infections in homosexual men

Aetiology

Although playing a small part in the global epidemiology of these infections, the sexual transmission of enteric pathogens amongst homosexual men is important. Oro-anal contact is the principal means of acquisition of these organisms that include bacteria (*Shigella* spp., *Salmonella* spp., *Campylobacter* spp.), viruses (hepatitis A, coronaviruses), protozoa (*Giardia intestinalis*, *Cryptosporidium parvum*, *Entamoeba histolytica*) and nematodes (*Enterobius vermicularis*). Symptomless carriers are important.

Clinical features

In immunocompetent men, the bacterial infections may be symptomless or cause an acute self-limiting diarrhoeal illness; in AIDS patients a more prolonged and severe illness may occur. A panproctocolitis is noted. Coronaviruses may be associated with diarrhoea and hepatitis A with acute icteric hepatitis. Although a proctocolitis with diarrhoea may result from *E. histolytica* infestation, most homosexual men are infested with a non-pathogenic stock of the amoeba *Entamoeba dispar*. *Giardia* affects the upper small intestine, sometimes producing diarrhoea with features of malabsorption. In immunocompetent individuals, infection with *C. parvum* results in a self-limiting diarrhoeal illness; immunocompromised patients may have persistent and often severe diarrhoea. Enterobiasis is often associated with pruritus ani.

Diagnosis

Diagnosis is achieved by the following approaches:
1. Bacterial infections by faecal cultures.
2. Hepatitis A by serology and coronaviruses by electron microscopy.
3. Protozoa by microscopy of faeces for cysts (Fig. 110), oocysts and trophozoites (Figs 111 & 112) (jejunal fluid and biopsy are sometimes used for diagnosis of giardiasis and *Cryptosporidium* infection).
4. *E. vermicularis* by sticky tape-strip microscopy (Fig. 113).

Treatment

Specific chemotherapy when indicated.

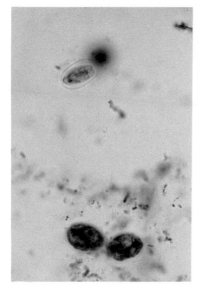

Fig. 110 Cysts of *G. intestinalis.*

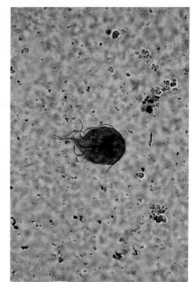

Fig. 111 Trophozoite of *G. intestinalis.*

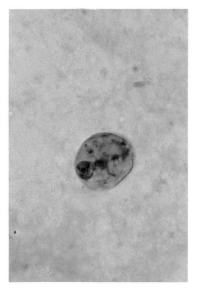

Fig. 112 Trophozoite of *E. histolytica.*

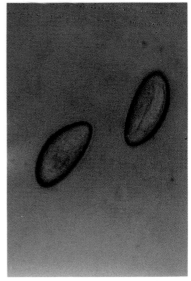

Fig. 113 Ova of *E. vermicularis.*

Aetiology | *Pthirus pubis* (crab louse) (Figs 114 & 115) infests the strong hairs of the pubic and perianal areas, those of the thighs, legs, forearms, axillae, chest and, less frequently, eyelashes, eyebrows and beard. Eggs (Fig. 116) are laid at the bases of the hairs and after hatching the nymphs undergo three moults before maturity is reached, usually 3 weeks from oviposition.

Epidemiology | *P. pubis* is transmitted by close contact, particularly during sexual intercourse. As the louse may survive away from the body for up to 24 h depending on conditions, transmission by fomites may rarely be possible.

Clinical features | Although many individuals are symptomless, pruritus in the pubic area is the most common feature. Rarely, bluish macules are seen on the trunk at the site of bites (maculae caeruleae). Pyoderma may result from scratching.

Treatment | Malathion (1%), carbaryl (1%) and phenothrin lotions are useful in that they are lethal to lice and eggs. Petroleum jelly applied twice daily is used to treat eyelash infestation.

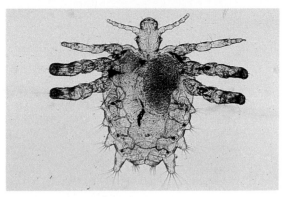

Fig. 114 *P. pubis* (adult female).

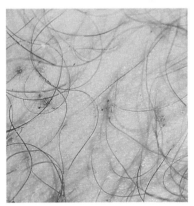

Fig. 115 Pthiriasis of pubic hair.

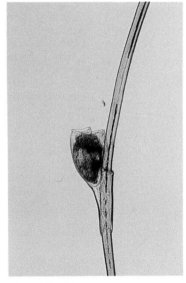

Fig. 116 *P. pubis* egg.

23 / Scabies

Aetiology	Caused by the mite *Sarcoptes scabiei* (Fig. 117) that burrows down into the stratum corneum where the female lays her eggs. These hatch and the larva leaves the burrow to find a new area of skin into which it burrows.
Epidemiology	Personal contact including sexual intercourse is the most usual means of acquisition of the parasite. Household spread is also recognised.
Clinical features	The patient develops itch, particularly on retiring at night 4–6 weeks after exposure, or earlier if there has been a previous infestation. The skin rash is roughly symmetrically distributed and is composed of burrows (Fig. 118), that may be found on the finger webs and sides of the digits, flexor surfaces of the wrists and the penis (Fig. 119), and papules that are seen on these areas and on the extensor surfaces of the elbows, anterior axillary folds, female breasts, abdomen, scrotum, lower buttocks and upper thighs. Papules may become excoriated and eczematous changes are common. Reddish-brown pruritic nodules that may persist for months even after treatment may be found on the elbows, axillary folds and male genitalia. In people who bathe frequently, lesions are often sparse. Secondary infection may occur.
Diagnosis	Mites and eggs found in skin scrapings.
Treatment	Malathion and permethrin are effective. The itch may persist for several weeks.

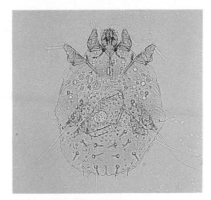

Fig. 117 Mite of *S. scabiei*.

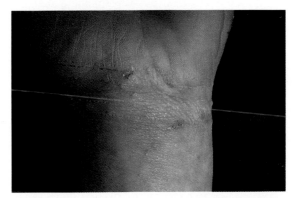

Fig. 118 Scabetic burrows.

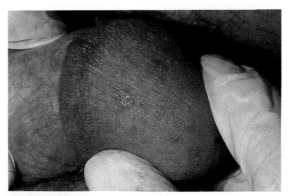

Fig. 119 Scabetic papules on the penis.

Aetiology	Syphilis is caused by the bacterium *Treponema pallidum* spp. *pallidum*, which is spread principally by sexual contact but which can be acquired congenitally.
Epidemiology	In the UK, the incidence of early syphilis fell sharply in the immediate post-war years and remained constant until the mid-1980s, when it fell further. (Prior to the advent of HIV infection, some 50% of male cases had been acquired homosexually, but with changing sexual behaviour of men who have sex with other men, few such cases are now reported). There continues to be an increase in the number of cases of early syphilis reported from eastern Europe. In the UK the incidence of late-stage and congenital infection remains low. Syphilis is still prevalent in the developing world. Although individuals with syphilis of more than 4 years' duration cease to be infectious sexually, a pregnant woman can transmit the infection at any stage to her child during the later stages of pregnancy.
Clinical features	**Acquired syphilis** *Primary syphilis* After a prepatent period of about 3 weeks (range 10–90 d), a dull red papule that soon ulcerates develops at the site of inoculation of the treponeme. The ulcer (chancre) is single, painless, and well-demarcated. It is indurated but not tender; the full, red, flat surface may be covered with a flat crust. Serous fluid but not blood exudes from the surface. The lesion may be found anywhere on the external genitalia (Figs 120 & 121) or on the cervix uteri. Anal chancres (Fig. 122) may be atypical and resemble fissures. Oral lesions are rare. Bilateral inguinal lymph node enlargement occurs. The lesion heals within 3–8 weeks, leaving a thin scar.

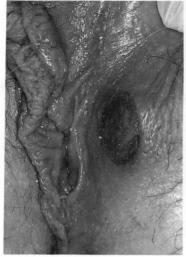

Fig. 120 Vulval chancre.

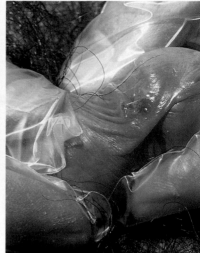

Fig. 121 Penile chancre.

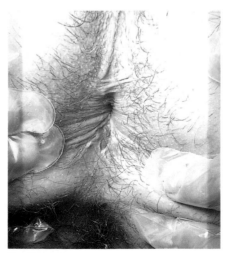

Fig. 122 Chancre of anal canal.

Acquired syphilis (contd)
Secondary syphilis
Signs of this stage develop 7–10 weeks after infection, and in some patients the primary lesion is still present. The clinical features may appear and regress at intervals over a 2-year period. The patient complains of malaise, mild fever, headache, a skin rash that may be mildly pruritic, hoarseness, swollen lymph nodes, patchy or diffuse hair loss, arthralgia and bone pain.

Skin lesions are noticed in over 80% of cases. The earliest lesions are rose-pink macules that are symmetrically distributed over the body (Fig. 123). A symmetrically distributed papular rash is more commonly seen (Figs 124 & 125). Initially the lesions have a shiny surface but later scaling occurs (Fig. 126). Papules may be found in the nasolabial folds, below the hairline, and on the palms of hands (Fig. 127, p. 94) and soles of feet. In moist areas such as the perianal region, the papules are hypertrophic and may be eroded (condylomata lata) (Fig. 128, p. 94). Involvement of the hair follicles may result in patchy hair loss (Fig. 129, p. 94). In the later stages of secondary syphilis the papules become fewer and are distributed asymmetrically. Condylomata lata may be the only feature at this stage. Lesions heal without scarring but depigmentation may occur.

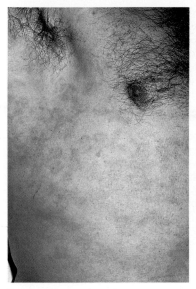

Fig. 123 Early macular rash.

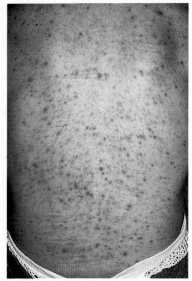

Fig. 124 Maculopapular rash.

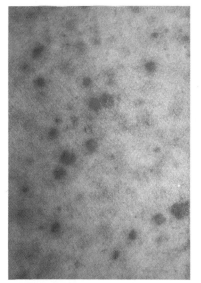

Fig. 125 Maculopapular rash (close up).

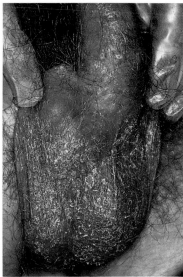

Fig. 126 Psoriasiform rash.

Acquired syphilis (contd)
Secondary syphilis (contd)

Mucosal lesions occur in 30% of patients. They are oval superficial ulcers covered with a grey membrane (Fig. 130); adjacent lesions may coalesce. They are found on the tonsils, buccal mucosa, tongue, larynx and genitalia.

Other features of secondary syphilis include generalised lymphadenopathy, and less commonly, hepatitis, glomerulonephritis, choroidoretinitis, meningoencephalitis, and periostitis.

The differential diagnosis of secondary syphilis includes drug eruptions, measles, rubella, infectious mononucleosis, pityriasis rosea, psoriasis, lichen planus, pityriasis lichenoides, anogenital warts, herpes simplex infection, trichophytides, aphthous ulceration and keratotic eczema.

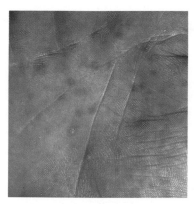

Fig. 127 Palmar lesions.

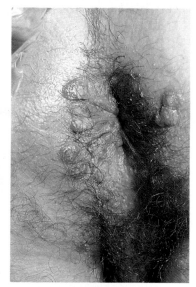

Fig. 128 Condylomata lata.

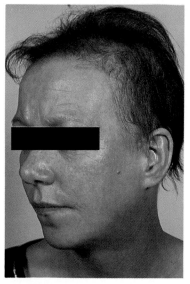

Fig. 129 Diffuse alopecia.

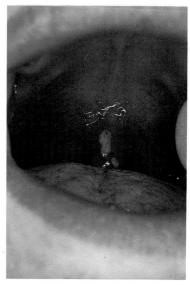

Fig. 130 Mucous patch.

Acquired syphilis (contd)

Latent syphilis

The lesions of secondary syphilis heal and the disease becomes latent, being detectable only by serological testing. The distinction between early-latent and late-latent disease is arbitrary, but syphilis of over 2 years' duration is considered to be in its late stages.

Gummatous syphilis

When host resistance to the treponeme fails in the late stages of infection, localised gummatous lesions (syphilitic granulation tissue) develop. The lesion is a single punched ulcer of the skin, especially of the scalp, upper outer aspect of the leg (Fig. 131) or the sternoclavicular region. The mouth or pharynx may be affected. Diffuse infiltration of the tongue with chronic superficial glossitis on which leukoplakia (Fig. 132) may subsequently develop may occur. Gummatous periostitis or osteitis may be features. Generally there is a good response to treatment.

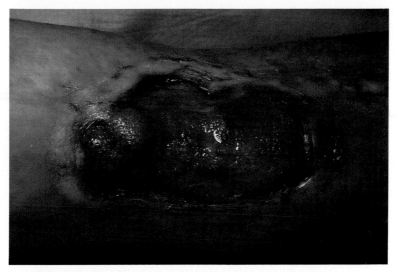

Fig. 131 Gumma of leg.

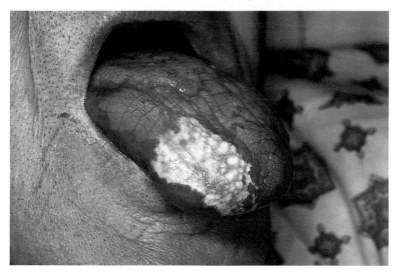

Fig. 132 Leukoplakia of tongue.

Acquired syphilis (contd)
Neurosyphilis
This may be symptomless and detectable only by the examination of the cerebrospinal fluid (CSF). The clinical course may be accelerated if there is concomitant HIV infection. Meningovascular syphilis may produce headache, cranial nerve palsies, and if the cerebral vessels are affected, focal signs and mental deterioration. General paralysis of the insane (GPI) can develop 7–15 years after infection; dementia is the usual presenting feature. In tabes dorsalis, the degenerative lesions are concentrated on the dorsal columns of the lumbosacral and lower thoracic levels of the spinal cord. Lightning pains, paraesthesiae, ataxia, disturbances of bladder and bowel control, and crises (paroxysmal painful disorders of the viscera) are all features. There is muscle hypotonia with diminution of lower limb reflexes, and optic atrophy. Trophic ulcers (Fig. 133) may develop on the soles of feet and neuropathic joints (Charcot's) (Fig. 134) may occur in the lower limbs.

The Argyll-Robertson pupil is the characteristic pupillary change in all forms of late neurosyphilis. It is small, constant in size, reacting to accommodation but not to light, patchily depigmented, and dilating slowly to mydriatics. Other abnormalities are also found.

Cardiovascular syphilis
Aortitis, especially of the aortic ring and ascending part of the aorta with resulting destruction of elastic tissue, may produce aortic incompetence or aneurysm formation (Fig. 135).

Congenital syphilis
T. pallidum can cross the placenta of an infected mother and produce early or late signs of infection. In view of the rarity of this condition in industrialised countries, the clinical features of congenital syphilis are not considered here.

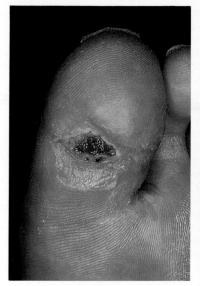

Fig. 133 Perforating ulcer.

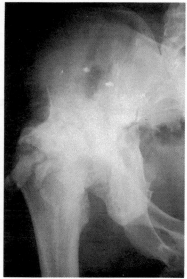

Fig. 134 Neuropathic (Charcot's) joint.

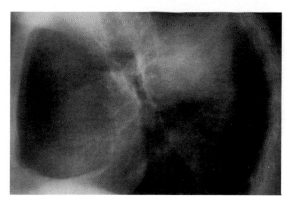

Fig. 135 Aortic aneurysm.

Diagnosis	*T. pallidum* can be detected in the serum from the base of a chancre by dark-field microscopy (Fig. 136) or direct immunofluorescence (Fig. 137). Serological tests form the principal diagnostic methods for all other stages of the infection. In many laboratories an enzyme immunoassay (EIA) has replaced the cardiolipid antibody tests (e.g. Venereal Diseases Research Laboratory (VDRL) test and the rapid plasma reagin (RPR) test and the *Treponema pallidum* haemagglutination (TPHA) test for screening. A positive result in the EIA (or in the TPHA/VDRL screening tests) is confirmed by testing with another specific treponemal test such as the fluorescent treponemal antibody absorption (FTA-Abs) test. The latter is also the most sensitive serological test for early disease. In untreated infections the EIA and TPHA tests may remain positive for life (IgG antibodies). Over time the VDRL becomes negative in one-third of cases. Specific IgM can be detected in untreated disease. With successful treatment, the VDRL becomes negative within about 1 year of treatment of early syphilis; the EIA, TPHA and FTA-Abs may remain positive for years. Persistence of cardiolipin and treponemal antibodies is common after treatment of late-stage disease. Neurosyphilis is diagnosed by finding treponemal antibodies in the CSF. The detection of 19S (IgM) antibodies in the baby's blood is the most reliable test for congenital infection. Serum from patients with the endemic treponematoses yields positive results in the above tests.
Treatment	Penicillin is the treatment of choice. In individuals with penicillin hypersensitivity, tetracyclines or erythromycin are alternatives. The Jarisch-Herxheimer reaction may occur within 4 h of treatment of early syphilis and neurosyphilis.

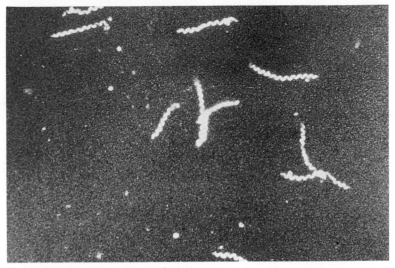

Fig. 136 *T. pallidum* detected by dark-field microscopy.

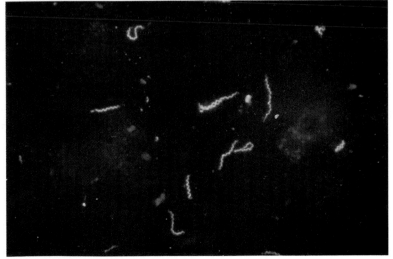

Fig. 137 *T. pallidum* detected by direct immunofluorescence.

Aetiology

Caused by *Haemophilus ducreyi*, this is an ulcerative condition of the genitalia that is found mostly in tropical countries.

Clinical features

Single or multiple painful, tender superficial ulcers develop within a week of exposure (Fig. 138). Phimosis may result from the inflammation. Inguinal lymph nodes on one or both sides enlarge and may suppurate, with the development of a unilocular abscess (bubo) (Fig. 139) that may rupture to form a sinus.

Diagnosis

The diagnosis is made by Gram-smear microscopy and culture of material from the edge of the ulcer.

Treatment

Azithromycin given orally or ceftriaxone given by i.m. injection are satisfactory treatments. Alternatively, a course of either ciprofloxacin or erythromycin can be used.

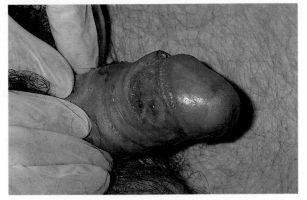

Fig. 138 Subpreputial chancroid.

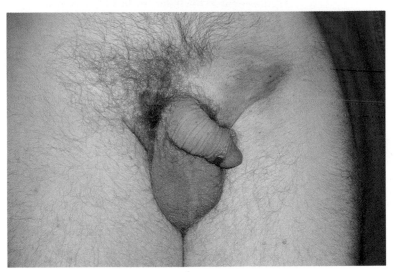

Fig. 139 Penile chancroid with bubo.

Aetiology

This is caused by the bacterium *Klebsiella granulomatis*. As it predominantly affects the genitalia, granuloma inguinale is thought to be sexually transmitted although this has not been proved conclusively. The condition is seen mainly in the tropics.

Clinical features

The prepatent period may be from 3 d to 6 months. The earliest lesion is a flat-topped papule that soon ulcerates. The ulcer spreads slowly along skin folds and the base may become elevated above the surrounding tissue (Figs 140 & 141). Extensive scarring occurs in some patients, especially women in whom vulval oedema occurs. Extra genital sites are sometimes affected. Cancer may supervene later.

Diagnosis

On Giemsa staining of ulcer tissue, the bacteria are seen in mononuclear cells as the so-called Donovan bodies (Fig. 142).

Treatment

This is usually with either tetracyclines or co-trimoxazole.

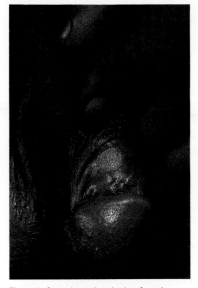

Fig. 140 Granuloma inguinale of penis.

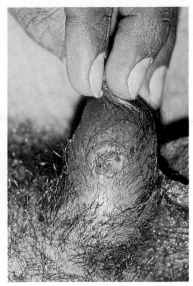

Fig. 141 Granuloma inguinale of penis.

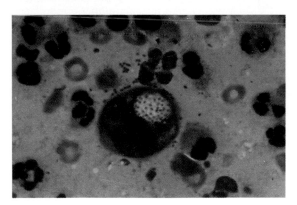

Fig. 142 Donovan bodies in a tissue smear.

27 / Lymphogranuloma venereum

Aetiology

Lymphogranuloma venereum (LGV) is caused by the L 1–3 serovars of *Chlamydia trachomatis*. Most cases are found in the tropics.

Clinical features

A primary lesion is noticed by only one-third of those infected. After 3 d to 3 weeks, the lesion begins as a small painless papule, which ulcerates (Fig. 143) and then heals after a few days. Thereafter, the patient develops tender, inguinal lymphadenopathy that is unilateral in two-thirds of cases. Abscesses (buboes) may form (Fig. 144), and these may rupture resulting in sinus formation. The development of multiple buboes above and below Roupart's ligament may give 'the sign of the groove'.

Anorectal infection may result in an acute ulcerative proctitis.

Chronic vulval ulceration (esthiomene) and genital elephantiasis are uncommon later complications.

Diagnosis

Culture for *C. trachomatis* may be attempted from aspirated bubo pus. Serological tests may also be used.

Treatment

Tetracyclines such as doxycycline are usually given. Alternatives are erythromycin and rifampicin. Buboes should be aspirated to prevent rupture and sinus formation.

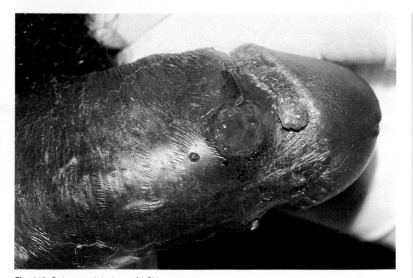

Fig. 143 Subpreputial ulcer of LGV.

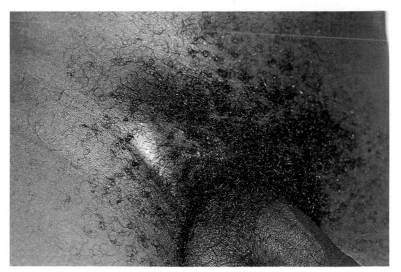

Fig. 144 Bubo of LGV.

Balanoposthitis

Common in uncircumcised men and sometimes caused by Streptococci (Fig. 145), it is more often associated with anaerobic infections (Fig. 146), but it can be a feature of contact dermatitis or allergic contact dermatitis. There is pain or itch, and often a malodorous subpreputial discharge. The inner surface of the prepuce and glans are reddened and there is a purulent discharge in the preputial sac. There may be superficial ulceration and preputial oedema with phimosis. Inguinal lymphadenitis is common.

Saline lavage is helpful and in more severe cases penicillin or metronidazole is needed. The urine must always be tested for glycosuria.

Tinea cruris

Caused by a species of dermatophyte, the lesions are bilateral and extend down the thighs and on to the scrotum (Fig. 147). The skin is reddened and scaly and the margins are sharp. Small satellite lesions are usual. Diagnosis is made by finding hyphae in KOH preparations of skin scrapings. Treatment is with a topical imidazole.

Erythrasma

Caused by *Corynebacterium minutissimum*, erythrasma presents as non-pruritic, irregularly shaped but sharply marginated red to brown patches that later become scaly.

Uni- or bilateral lesions affect the thighs and scrotum. Topical imidazoles are effective.

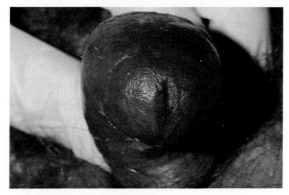

Fig. 145 Streptococcal balanoposthitis.

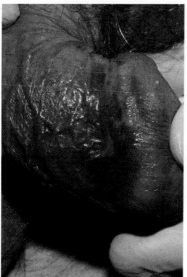

Fig. 146 Anaerobic balanoposthitis.

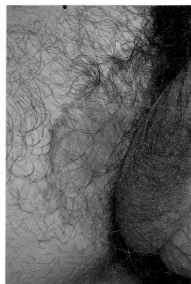

Fig. 147 Tinea cruris.

Psoriasis
Papules with scaling may be seen on the glans penis (Fig. 148) of the circumcised male. In the uncircumcised male, the lesions are red with well-defined edges but there is no scaling. Other features are usually found, e.g. pitting of the nails. Diffuse plaques in the genitocrural folds or perianal region (Fig. 149) are red and sharply defined.

Lichen planus
Violaceous papules with flat shiny surfaces, less than 1mm to more than 1cm may be found on the external genitalia. Often symptomless, they may be pruritic. Linear lesions occur at the site of scratching and annular lesions are common on the penis (Fig. 150). Lesions are self-limiting. In the buccal mucosa there may be a network of white streaks.

Eczema
The external genitalia may be involved in widespread eczema. Seborrhoeic dermatitis is usually flexural, the area being reddened with well-defined edges. Areas of lichenification (*lichen simplex*) (Fig. 151) may result from prolonged rubbing.

Irritant dermatitis
Painful reddened lesions with swelling and ulceration may follow contact with chemicals.

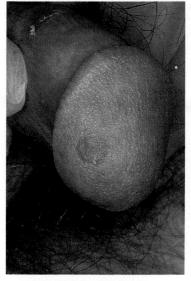

Fig. 148 Psoriasis of glans penis.

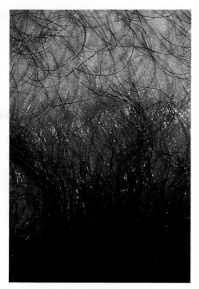

Fig. 149 Psoriasis of perianal region.

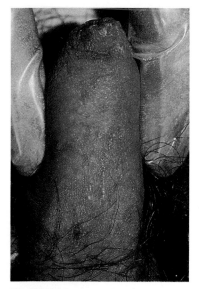

Fig. 150 Lichen planus of penis.

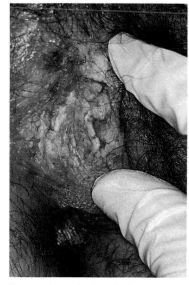

Fig. 151 Lichen simplex of vulva.

Lichen sclerosus et atrophicus

Lichen sclerosus et atrophicus (LSA) is rare and affects women more frequently than men. The median age at onset is about 50 years in women and slightly earlier in men.

Clinical features

Vulval soreness and dyspareunia are the symptoms in females. The perianal region, inner aspects of the labia minora and vestibule are usually affected. Pearly-white atrophic papules with follicular plugging may be seen in the perianal region but on the vulva (Fig. 152) friction and moisture produce erosion of their surfaces resulting in a red, raw area. There is genital atrophy and the introitus is constricted. Haemorrhagic vesicles and telangiectatic lesions are common. Lichenification and small, deep fissures may result. Lesions may be found elsewhere on the body.

The glans penis and prepuce (Fig. 153) are the sites affected in the male. Phimosis is a feature and meatal stricture may ensue. The glans and mucosal surface of the prepuce are white, the surface often showing telangiectasia.

When the onset has been in middle age, the lesions are unlikely to remit. Leukoplakia and squamous cell carcinoma may complicate the condition.

Treatment

The treatment is symptomatic with bland creams or corticosteroid preparations. In the male there should be attention to hygiene. Circumcision and urethral meatotomy may be necessary.

Plasma cell balanitis

Of uncertain cause, this presents in older men as a chronic balanitis with a moist shiny surface stippled with 'cayenne pepper' spots. There is a poor response to any treatment.

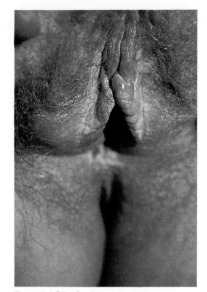

Fig. 152 LSA of vulva.

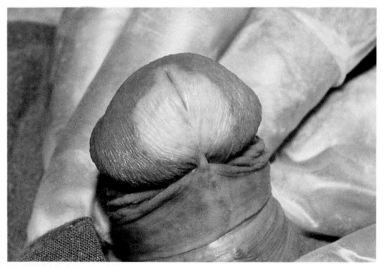

Fig. 153 LSA of penis.

Bullous erythema multiforme

Aetiology

Also known as Stevens–Johnson syndrome. This can be associated with viral (especially herpes simplex) and bacterial (especially *Mycoplasma pneumoniae*) infections, drugs (such as sulphonamides) and collagen diseases. In more than 50% of cases there is no detectable precipitating factor.

Clinical features

Bullae develop suddenly on the oral (Fig. 154) and genital (Fig. 155) mucosae, ulcerate and become covered with a greyish white membrane; haemorrhagic crusting is common. There may be a marked conjunctivitis. Skin lesions (Fig. 156) that are not always present are dull-red maculopapules that may develop into target lesions; cropping at intervals of a few days is usual. The rash is found on the hands, wrists, forearms, elbows and knees.

Treatment

Treatment is symptomatic, but corticosteroids may be needed in severe cases. Recurrences can occur, particularly with herpetic infections.

Fixed drug eruption

These lesions recur in the same site each time the particular drug is given. The glans penis is a common site (Fig. 157). There is an erythematous plaque that later darkens and is often surmounted by a bulla. Healing is accompanied by crusting and scaling. Residual pigmentation is common. Drugs that may be responsible include tetracycline, sulphonamides and barbiturates. ▶

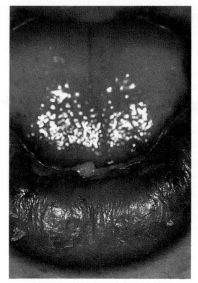

Fig. 154 Oral lesions of bullous erythema multiforme.

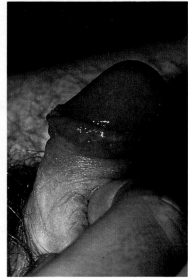

Fig. 155 Penile lesions of bullous erythema multiforme.

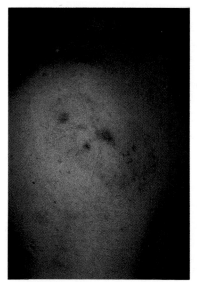

Fig. 156 Skin lesions of bullous erythema multiforme.

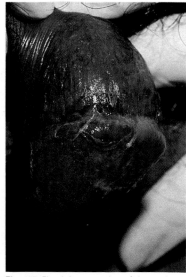

Fig. 157 Fixed drug eruption of the penis.

Pyoderma gangrenosum

This condition can be associated with ulcerative colitis, rheumatoid arthritis and chronic suppurative conditions. The characteristic lesion is an irregular ulcer with a ragged, bluish and overhanging edge, and a necrotic base (Figs 158 & 159). Multiple ulcers are sometimes found. Treatment is symptomatic, but the ulceration can persist for years. Any underlying condition should be treated.

Crohn's disease

This may affect the anogenital region and present as vulval oedema, oedematous perianal skin tags, fistulae, abscesses and ulceration (Fig. 160). Diagnosis is by histology. Differential diagnosis includes tuberculosis, lymphogranuloma venereum, malignancy, hidradenitis and deep fungal infection.

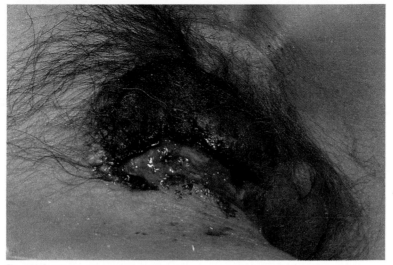

Fig. 158 Pyoderma gangrenosum of the vulva.

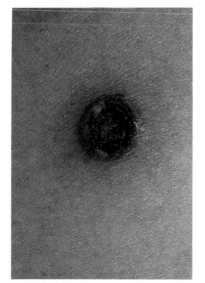

Fig. 159 Pyoderma gangrenosum of the thigh.

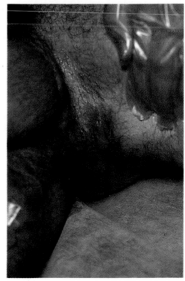

Fig. 160 Perianal Crohn's disease, showing sinuses.

Behçets' syndrome

This is a multisystem disease characterised by oral, genital and ocular lesions with a tendency to exacerbations and remissions. It is of unknown aetiology but principally affects individuals of east Mediterranean or Japanese origin. The common histological feature is a vasculitis.

Clinical features

In the mucocutaneous form of the syndrome, there are recurrent multiple, painful ulcers of the oral mucosa (Fig. 161). The lesions usually heal within 2 weeks but some may be persistent and heal with scarring. Similar ulceration of the genitalia may occur (Figs 162 & 163). Skin lesions include ulceration, pustules, erythema nodosum and erythema multiforme. The mucocutaneous signs may be the only features of Behçets' syndrome or may accompany or antedate other manifestations. Anterior uveitis, phlebitis, venous occlusion, macular or optic-disc oedema and vitreous cellular infiltration are the ocular features; blindness may result. In about 50% of cases, arthritis or arthralgia of the knees, ankles, wrists and elbows occurs. Neurological features include cranial nerve palsies, cerebellar and spinal cord lesions and meningoencephalitis.

Treatment

Oral and genital ulceration may respond to treatment with topical corticosteroids but ocular and visceral disease may require immunosuppressive chemotherapy. Thalidomide may be helpful in those with troublesome recurrent oral or genital ulceration.

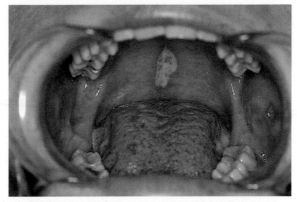

Fig. 161 Aphthous ulceration of mouth in Behets' syndrome.

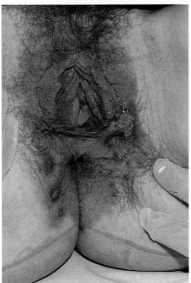

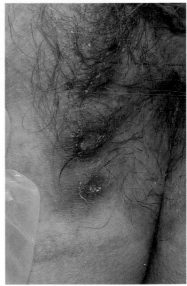

Fig. 162 Deep aphthous ulceration of vulva in Behcets' syndrome.

Fig. 163 Deep aphthous ulceration of vulva in Behcets' syndrome.

Intraepidermal carcinoma (Bowen's disease)
Middle-aged women are most commonly affected. The condition may progress to squamous cell carcinoma and be associated with malignancy elsewhere in the genital tract.

Pruritus vulvae or ani, or soreness are the symptoms. There is a well-demarcated red, slightly scaly and somewhat elevated plaque (Fig. 164) that slowly increases in size. Any part of the vulva can be involved. The diagnosis is made by histology. Surgical excision or topical application of 5-fluorouracil are used to treat the condition.

Erythroplasia of Queyrat
This premalignant condition occurs in men aged between 50 and 60 years. There is a very slightly elevated, soft, well-demarcated, bright-red velvety plaque that occurs on the glans penis or mucosal surface of the prepuce (Fig. 165). It is slowly progressive. The diagnosis is made by biopsy. Treatment is by cryotherapy or the topical application of 5-fluorouracil.

Squamous cell carcinoma
On the penis the most common presentation is that of a warty lesion in the preputial sac (Fig. 166); ulceration may occur later. Rarely, the locally invasive form (Buschke-Lowenstein) may occur. Vulval (Fig. 167) and anal lesions tend to be ulcerated. Other malignancies such as basal cell carcinoma and melanoma are rare.

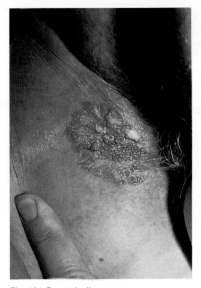

Fig. 164 Bowen's disease.

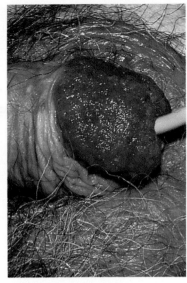

Fig. 165 Erythroplasia of Queyrat.

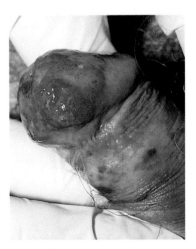

Fig. 166 Squamous cell carcinoma of penis.

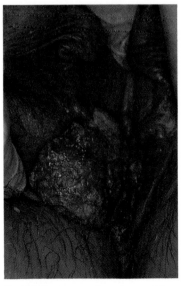

Fig. 167 Squamous cell carcinoma of the vulva.

Index